CONTENTS

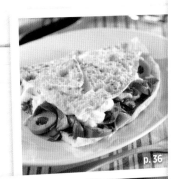

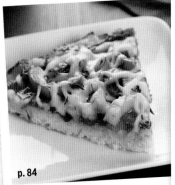

p. 36

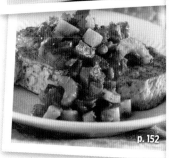

p. 84

p. 152

INTRODUCTION

DIETARY FATS AND OILS, WEIGHT AND HEALTH

Want to hear some good news about dietary fats and oils—especially how they relate to weight and health?

Consuming dietary fats and oils is not as bad as you might think—nor will consuming dietary fats and oils necessarily make you fat. The right amounts and types of dietary fats and oils may actually be satisfying and contribute to weight loss and weight maintenance. Dietary fats and oils are essential to your overall diet. Understanding what dietary fats and oils are and how they fit into an overall diet will help you with food selection, preparation and meal and menu planning.

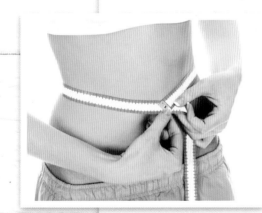

A diet that is based on ketones (organic compounds that are produced when dietary carbohydrates are limited), ketosis is a normal metabolic process whereby the body burns stored fats instead of glucose from carbohydrates for energy. A diet based on ketosis, with its abundance of dietary fats and oils may actually help your dieting efforts. Understanding more about ketones and their place in a ketogenic diet may assist your food choices and dietary efforts.

In addition to their role in weight loss and weight management, different types of dietary fats and oils and ketones are important for brain function, some disease protection and management, and overall health if used advantageously and correctly.

Dietary fats and oils are naturally found in foods and beverages such as dairy products, eggs, nuts, meats and seeds. Manufactured dietary fats and oils are found in some beverages, processed foods like margarine, cheeses and meats. Ketones are produced by the human body—you'll soon discover how.

There are differing viewpoints on the benefits of different types of dietary fats and oils and about ketones, the ideal amounts to consume and how ketones may sensibly be used for weight loss.

The purpose of this book is to help educate you about the types of dietary and blood fats and their contribution to health, and their relation to ketones and the ketogenic diet. It provides you with recipes that focus on healthy fats, proteins and non-starchy vegetables and de-emphasizes carbohydrates—particularly those that are refined or processed.

Your healthcare provider may help you determine if these approaches to eating and dieting are appropriate for you, so ask your doctor before you begin this or any other diet program.

CHOOSE THE RIGHT FATS

Fats are essential for proper body functioning and contribute satisfaction to diets, plus fats add flavor to foods and beverages. Still, fats provide more than twice the number of calories as carbohydrates or proteins (9 calories per gram compared to four calories per gram respectively). On a ketogenic diet, there is a different approach to fats than other diets that may restrict fats. The key is to understand the importance of fats in ketogenic diets and how to use them to your advantage.

TYPES OF FATS

Saturated fats are primarily found in foods from animal sources, such as meat, poultry and full-fat dairy products, while trans fats are mostly created when oils are partially hydrogenated to improve their cooking applications and to give them a longer shelf life. Saturated and trans fats may place a person at greater risk for heart disease. On the other hand, unsaturated fats that include monounsaturated and polyunsaturated fatty acids, found in plant-based foods such as avocados, nuts and seeds and olives and olive oil, and in fatty fish such as salmon, sardines and tuna tend to lower the risk of heart issues.

The American Heart Association (AHA) Diet and Lifestyle Recommendations suggest that a person limit saturated and trans fats and replace them with monounsaturated and polyunsaturated fats. If blood cholesterol needs to be lowered, then the recommendation is to reduce saturated fat to no more than 5 to 6 percent of total calories. For someone consuming 2,000 calories a day, this is about 13 grams of saturated fat, or about 117 calories. This is the equivalent of about 1 ounce of Cheddar cheese (9.4% total fat with 6 grams of saturated fat) and about 3 ounces of regular ground beef (25% total fat with 6.1 grams of saturated fat).

Try to eliminate trans fats (fats that have been processed into saturated fats) completely, or limit them to less than 1 percent of total daily calories. On a 2,000-calorie diet, this means that fewer than 20 calories (about 2 grams) should be derived from trans fats.

> THE KEY IS TO UNDERSTAND THE IMPORTANCE OF FATS IN KETOGENIC DIETS AND HOW TO USE THEM TO YOUR ADVANTAGE.

In contrast, in the ketogenic diet as much as 75 percent of daily calories are derived from fat; up to 30 percent of daily calories are to come from proteins and no more than 10 percent of daily calories are to come from carbohydrates (about 20 to 50 grams).

WHAT'S INSIDE FATS AND OILS?

Fats and oils are composed of fatty acids that contain different properties. Some fatty acids are considered unhealthy and may contribute to certain diseases, while other fatty acids are considered to be healthier and may be better for weight loss and weight maintenance in the long run.

The main types of fatty acids that are found in our food supply include saturated fatty acids, monounsaturated fatty acids, polyunsaturated fatty acids, trans fatty acids, omega-3 and omega-6 fatty acids and triglycerides. Cholesterol is a waxy substance that is found in some foods and beverages and is also produced by the body.

Saturated fatty acids (or saturated fats) are solid at room temperature. They are fully saturated or packed with fatty acids. (The name refers to its chemical makeup; saturated fats are short-chain fats with no double bonds and are "saturated" or filled with hydrogen.) They are a hard type of fat for the body to break down and may increase the risk for heart disease and stroke.

Saturated fats are mostly found in animal foods such as dairy products, lard and meats and in some tropical oils including coconut, palm and palm kernel oil. By consuming a mixture of foods and beverages that are higher in saturated fatty acids, monounsaturated fatty acids and omega-3 fatty acids, blood cholesterol levels may be lowered and blood profiles may improve. An active lifestyle is also a contributing factor in improved lipid profiles.

Monounsaturated fatty acids (or monounsaturated fats) are liquid or soft at room temperature. They have one space or opening within their chain of fatty acids, which makes it easier for the body to metabolize or break down. Partly for this reason, monounsaturated fats are considered to be healthier than saturated fats. Also, monounsaturated fats may help to lower blood cholesterol and decrease the risk of heart disease, so they are considered to be "heart-healthy".

Monounsaturated fats are found in avocados, canola oil, olives and nuts and their respective oils, seeds, and safflower and sunflower oils. They are more fragile than saturated fatty acids and may break down with exposure to air or heat.

Polyunsaturated fatty acids (or polyunsaturated fats) may also be liquid or soft at room temperature, but they may solidify when chilled. Polyunsaturated fats have many spaces or openings within their chain of fatty acids, which makes them much easier for the body to process (and to breakdown with exposure to air or heat).

Polyunsaturated fats provide nutrients for the development and maintenance of healthy body cells, which include vitamin E, an important antioxidant that protects the cells from damage. Polyunsaturated fats may also help to reduce blood cholesterol and lower the risk of heart disease and stroke when they are consumed in moderation and when they replace saturated and trans fats in the diet. Daily fat consumption should be comprised mostly of monounsaturated or polyunsaturated fats.

> **DAILY FAT CONSUMPTION SHOULD BE COMPRISED MOSTLY OF MONOUNSATURATED OR POLYUNSATURATED FATS.**

Oils with polyunsaturated fats include corn, olive, soybean and sunflower oils. Polyunsaturated fats may also be found in fatty fish including herring, mackerel, salmon and trout, along with other seafood, nuts and seeds. By reducing highly processed carbohydrate-containing foods in the diet, some polyunsaturated fats will be reduced, but those from healthier food sources should remain.

Trans fatty acids (or trans fats) are fatty acids that have been processed into saturated fats. Trans fats are created by industrial methods through the process of hydrogenation, which solidifies or partially solidifies liquid vegetable oils. Trans fats, difficult for the body to process and eliminate, trigger inflammation. Consequently, trans fats are implicated in cardiovascular disease, diabetes, insulin resistance, metabolic disease and stroke.

Trans fats are commonly found in many fried foods and baked goods such as crackers, cookies, chips, French fries, pastries, pie crust and pizza dough. They also naturally occur in small amounts in some dairy products and meats.

The terms "hydrogenated" and "partially hydrogenated oils" on the Nutrition Facts Panel used to mean that foods and beverages contained trans fats. In 2015, the U.S. Food and Drug Administration (FDA) determined that partially hydrogenated oils (the primary dietary source of artificial trans fats in processed foods) are "generally not recognized as safe in human food." Food manufacturers were given 3 years (until 2018) to comply with removing all trans fats from food.

Inspect nutrition labels to make sure you're avoiding all trans fats. Even if a food package states "0 grams of trans fats," it might still contain some trans fats if the amount per serving is less than 0.5 grams, so check the ingredients to make sure there are no hydrogenated or partially hydrogenated oils listed.

Omega-3 and **omega-6 fatty acids** are both types of polyunsaturated fats with unique properties.

Omega-3 fatty acids (or omega-3 fats) are essential fats, which means that they must be supplied by the diet for healthy body functioning. Omega-3 fats, particularly EPA and DHA, are beneficial to the heart. They may decrease arrhythmias (abnormal heartbeats) and triglycerides stored in fat cells, increase tissue flexibility, improve cholesterol profiles, lower blood pressure, reduce inflammation and slow the growth of plaque in the arteries. (Plaque is a hard substance that is composed of cholesterol, calcium and clotting materials.)

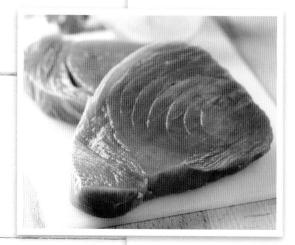

Omega-3 fats may also help to relieve the symptoms of chronic diseases such as arthritis, depression and dementia. EPA and DHA are components of hormones that regulate immune function and DHA is vital for brain development and cognition.

Good sources of omega-3 fats include seafood such as mackerel, sardines, salmon, tuna and shellfish and plant sources like canola and soybean oils, flaxseed and walnuts.

Omega-6 fatty acids (or omega-6 fats) are also polyunsaturated fats and essential fatty acids. Omega-6 fats perform vital roles in brain function, normal development and growth. They also help maintain reproduction, regulate metabolism and support healthy skin and hair and bone health. However, omega-6 fatty acids may promote inflammation and contribute to complex regional pain syndrome. Chronic inflammation may contribute to asthma, autoimmunity and neurodegenerative diseases, cancers and coronary heart disease.

Omega-6 fats are prevalent in eggs, meats, poultry, salad dressings and corn, grape seed and sunflower oils. Linoleic acid (LA) is found in corn, cottonseed, safflower, soybean and sunflower oils among other oils. Arachidonic acid (AA) is found in small amounts in eggs, meats and poultry. LA can be converted to AA in the body. Omega-6 fats are often used in fried and processed foods, so a diet that is filled with highly processed foods may be disproportionately high in omega-6 fatty acids.

A healthy diet contains a balance of omega-3 and omega-6 fatty acids (or a ratio of 1:1), although the typical American diet tends to contain more omega-6 fatty acids than omega-3 fatty acids. Consuming more omega-3 fats through food sources, such as fish and chia or flaxseeds, may help to balance this pattern.

Cholesterol is an essential component in the cell membranes of brain and nerve cells and for hormone formation. It is used to maintain brain health for memory formation and for the production of hormones and vitamin D. When your skin absorbs sunlight, cholesterol within the cells is converted to vitamin D.

Cholesterol is a waxy substance that is found in animal foods such as dairy products, eggs and meats. The body produces cholesterol on its own from saturated fat or glucose so it is not needed from food.

Common thought used to be that a high level of dietary cholesterol contributed to coronary heart disease, diabetes, stroke or peripheral vascular disease. This is because excess cholesterol may form plaque between the layers of the artery walls. In turn, plaque may clog arteries, reduce their flexibility, interfere with blood circulation and lead to atherosclerosis, or "hardening" of the arteries. Plaque can also break apart and lead to blood clots. If blood clots form and block narrowed arteries, then a heart attack or stroke may occur.

Current thinking focuses more on the type of dietary and blood cholesterol and the types of fatty acids that they transport, and that consuming cholesterol doesn't necessarily lead to higher blood cholesterol levels. In fact, blood cholesterol levels may actually lower on a ketogenic diet.

There are two main types of cholesterol: **low-density lipoprotein (LDL)-cholesterol** (considered to be "bad" cholesterol) and **high-density lipoprotein (HDL)-cholesterol** (considered to be "good" cholesterol).

LDL-cholesterol is considered to be "bad" cholesterol because it may contribute to increased plaque in arteries, decrease flexibility and raise the risk of atherosclerosis (hardening of the arteries). Excess calories, dietary cholesterol, saturated fat, trans fats and total fat in the diet are some of the dietary factors that may increase LDL-cholesterol. Lifestyle factors and genetics that may also increase LDL-cholesterol include age, diabetes, family history, high blood pressure, male gender, obesity and physical inactivity. A healthy range of LDL-cholesterol is considered to be 100-129 mg/dL. Carbohydrate consumption from refined carbohydrates that are high in sugar and low in fiber is associated with higher levels of LDL-cholesterol and triglycerides. There is some thought that the size of LDL-particles are more important. Small and dense LDL particles may conveniently lodge in artery walls, cause inflammation and lead to heart disease.

HDL-cholesterol is considered to be "good" cholesterol because it helps remove cholesterol from the arteries and transport it back to the liver where it is broken down and excreted from the body. A healthy level of HDL-cholesterol (60 mg/dL or higher) may also protect against heart attack and stroke, while a low level of HDL-cholesterol (less than 40 mg/dL) may increase the risk of heart disease.

The protective benefits of HDL-cholesterol may depend upon the levels of other blood fats that are associated with coronary heart disease. For example, if LDL-cholesterol is not within normal range or if most LDL-cholesterol particles are small, even a high HDL-cholesterol level may not be protective.

Fish and soy foods, rich in mono and polyunsaturated fatty acids (MUFAs and PUFAs) may increase HDL-cholesterol, Consuming foods that are high in fiber and antioxidants from permissible ketogenic fruits and vegetables may help prevent LDL-cholesterol from injuring the artery walls.

Triglycerides are the main form of fat that is found in food and within the body. Triglycerides are composed of three fatty acids that vary in composition (saturated, unsaturated or a combination). High levels of triglycerides in the blood are associated with atherosclerosis. Certain diseases (such as diabetes or heart disease) and medications, cigarette smoking, excessive alcohol consumption, high carbohydrate intake, overweight and obesity, physical inactivity, smoking and some genetic disorders may contribute to elevated blood triglycerides.

This is because elevated blood triglycerides are often associated with high blood cholesterol, high LDL-cholesterol and/or low HDL-cholesterol, which are high-risk factors that are associated with these diseases and conditions.

COMMON FAT–CONTAINING FOODS

Common fat-containing foods include (but are not limited to) avocados, beef, butter, cheese, chocolate, coconut, coconut milk and coconut oil, nuts and seeds (including chia and flax seeds), oils (including canola, olive and peanut oils), salmon, sardines and walnuts.

AVOCADOS

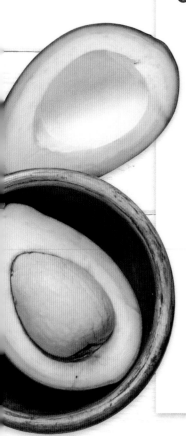

Avocados, technically a fruit, contain a lot of fat, but don't avoid them because of it! They contain omega-3 fatty acids, monounsaturated fatty acids, protein and fiber, as well as the B-vitamins, vitamin C, E and K, magnesium, potassium and healthy monounsaturated fatty acids. One cup of sliced avocado contains about 234 calories, 21 grams of total fat, 3.1 grams of saturated fat, 14 grams of monounsaturated fat and 2.7 grams of polyunsaturated fat with no cholesterol.

BEEF

Beef is more than burgers and steaks. There are three cuts: lean (3 grams of fat per ounce as round, sirloin and flank steak), medium-fat (5 grams of fat per ounce as rump roast, Porterhouse or T-bone) and high-fat (8 grams fat per ounce as USDA Prime, ribs and corned beef). Some cuts have polyunsaturated fats and others contain omega-3 fats and vitamins such as vitamins A and E, depending on their feed. Free-range beef might be rich in certain minerals from grazing. Beef is full of other nutrients, such as B-vitamins, choline, iron, protein, selenium and zinc and has prominence in ketogenic diets.

BUTTER AND MARGARINE

Butter has short, medium and long-chain fatty acids. The short-chain fatty acid is called butyric acid and the medium-chain fatty acid is called myristic acid. Both of these saturated fats have healthy benefits. They are relatively easy to transport and absorb by the body and they help supply flavor. In comparison, stearic and palmitic acids, the longer-chain fatty acids may be cardiovascular risk factors in higher amounts in the diet.

Margarine is an imitation butter spread that is manufactured from refined vegetable oil and water. Historically, vegetable oil was hardened in a process called hydrogenation that created unhealthy trans fats that contributed to heart disease. Trans fats have subsequently been removed from the majority of margarine products.

Margarine contains coloring, flavoring, milk solids, preservatives and sodium. The calories in margarine and butter may be similar in comparative portion sizes, but the composition of fatty acids differ. Generally, firmer margarines contain more saturated fats, while softer margarine may contain 10 to 20 percent saturated fats.

CHEESE

Cheese that is made from cow's milk contains about 69 percent saturated fatty acids, 24 percent monounsaturated fatty acids and 3 percent polyunsaturated fatty acids. Cheese that is made from goat's milk contains about 71 percent saturated fatty acids, 22 percent monounsaturated fatty acids and 3 percent polyunsaturated fatty acids. Cheddar, Swiss and Parmesan cheese are some varieties with the least total carbohydrates. Use cheese to add taste, texture and healthy fats to recipes.

CHOCOLATE

The fat that is found in cocoa plants and predominant in dark chocolate is cocoa butter, which is about 33 percent monounsaturated oleic fatty acid and 33 percent stearic fatty acid. In general, stearic fatty acids from plants, although saturated, seem to neither lower high HDL-cholesterol nor increase LDL- or total cholesterol. But on a ketogenic diet, be careful about the carbohydrates in chocolate in the forms of milk solids, sugars and others.

COCONUT, COCONUT MILK AND COCONUT OIL

Coconut, coconut milk and coconut oil are used throughout the world for their distinctive tastes and textures. They were considered unhealthy due to their saturated fat content but are now valued for their healthful properties.

About 60 percent of the saturated fats in coconut oil are in the form of medium-chain triglycerides (MCTs) that are absorbed directly by the gastro-intestinal tract and metabolized immediately by the liver for energy. For this and other reasons, MCTs may be beneficial in preventing atherosclerosis. MCTs may also help to trigger ketosis and may be effective for providing energy at the start of ketogenic diets.

Natural cholesterol-free coconut oil is solid at room temperature but it turns liquid at relatively low temperatures about (80°F). It can be substituted for cholesterol-containing butter or lard in cooking and baking. Two main types of coconut oil are refined and virgin; both are acceptable for cooking and baking, but virgin coconut oil has more a coco-nutty flavor than refined.

There are many liquid coconut products available; they cannot generally be used interchangeably. Their carbohydrate content may be too high to include in a ketogenic diet, so check the label. Coconut milk is made by simmering shredded coconut in water and then straining out and squeezing the coconut to extract the liquid. Coconut milk beverages may act as milk substitutes. Coconut water is the liquid from the inside of a coconut and is sold for drinking, not cooking. Coconut cream is similar to coconut milk, but is thicker because it contains less water. Often a layer of coconut cream will separate from the milk in a can of regular coconut milk. To blend it back into the milk, shake the can before opening. Or just pour the entire contents of the can into whatever you're cooking and stir well (the heat will melt the cream back into the milk). Avoid cream of coconut; this is sweetened coconut cream and it used primarily in desserts and drinks.

NUTS AND SEEDS

Nuts and seeds range in total fat, fatty acids and other nutrients. They are filled with protein, mostly mono-and polyunsaturated fatty acids and omega-3 fatty

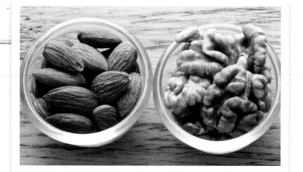

acids, insoluble fiber, the B vitamins and vitamin E and magnesium, manganese, phosphorus and zinc among other nutrients.

The fatty acids in almonds and walnuts may actually be helpful in lowering other blood fats. Almonds have been shown to help increase antioxidant vitamin E and lower blood cholesterol. Walnuts have a high percentage of omega-3 fats. Additionally, many nuts have a low Glycemic Index (GI) value, which means that they may be useful in insulin management and a good snack.

Pine nuts, common to heart-healthy Mediterranean diets, add a distinctive buttery and creamy touch to recipes. One-half cup contains about 673 calories, 10 grams of protein, 78 grams of total fat, 7 grams of saturated fat, almost 45 grams of monounsaturated fat, 24 grams of polyunsaturated fat and no cholesterol. The amount of dietary fiber ranges from 7 to 12 grams per half cup.

CHIA SEEDS

Chia seeds are tiny black seeds that contain antioxidants, calcium, carbohydrates, fats, fiber, omega-3 fatty acids and protein. Their fiber and omega-3 fat content are impressive with 11 grams of fiber per ounce (about 35 percent) and 60 percent of their total fat as ALA omega-3 fatty acids. Chia seeds are mild and nutty and add texture to foods and beverages. When mixed with water, chia seeds swell and become gel-like.

FLAX SEEDS

Similar to walnuts, flax seeds contain a significant amount of omega-3 fats such as alpha-linolenic acid (ALA): 1 tablespoon of ground flaxseed contains about 1.8 grams of omega-3 fats. Flax seeds also contain lignans with antioxidant and estrogen qualities and soluble and insoluble fibers that may offer protection against certain cancers and heart disease through their anti-inflammatory activity and heart beat normalization. Flax seeds and ground flaxseed spoil quickly so keep them in the freezer if you're not going to use them right away.

OILS

Like butter and margarine, some oils are also considered controversial—particularly the tropical oils: coconut oil, palm oil and palm kernel oil. Palm oil is an all-purpose cooking oil that is used in vegetable oil blends to impart flavor. It contains about 51 percent saturated fatty acids, 39 percent monounsaturated fatty acids and 10 percent polyunsaturated fatty acids. One tablespoon of palm oil contains about 5 grams of heart-healthy monounsaturated fatty acids.

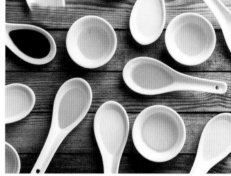

Palm kernel oil contains about 86 percent saturated fatty acids, 12 percent monounsaturated fatty acids and 2 percent polyunsaturated fatty acids. One tablespoon of palm kernel oil contains about 3.1 grams of heart-healthy monounsaturated fatty acids. Palm kernel oil is used in commercial baking since it tends to remains stable at high temperatures and can be stored longer than some other oils.

In contrast, canola oil, olive oil and peanut oil have more favorable fatty acid profiles. Canola oil contains about 6 percent saturated fatty acids, 62 percent monounsaturated fatty acids and 32 percent polyunsaturated fatty acids. One tablespoon of canola oil contains about 9 grams of heart-healthy monounsaturated fatty acids. Canola oil is commonly used for baking, frying and in salad dressings.

Olive oil contains about 14 percent saturated fatty acids, 73 percent monounsaturated fatty acids and 11 percent polyunsaturated fatty acids. One tablespoon of olive oil contains about 10 grams of heart-healthy monounsaturated fatty acids. Virgin olive oil is used as an all-purpose cooking oil and in salad dressing. Extra virgin olive oil is primarily used to dress salads, vegetables and entrées. Light and extra-light olive oil generally have less flavor and are mainly used for sautéing and stir-frying since they withstand more heat than extra virgin olive oil.

Peanut oil contains about 18 percent saturated fatty acids, 49 percent monounsaturated fatty acids and 33 percent polyunsaturated fatty acids. One tablespoon of peanut oil contains about 6 grams of heart-healthy monounsaturated fatty acids. Peanut oil has a higher smoke point than most olive oil blends, so is useful as an all-purpose oil in cooking and frying. Peanut oil is commonly used in Asian cuisine, while olive oil is used in Mediterranean cuisine. Canola oil is an all-purpose oil used in all types of cooking.

SALMON, SARDINES AND OTHER FATTY FISH

Generally the amount of omega-3 fatty acids in cold-water fatty fish, such as Albacore tuna, anchovies, Artic char, black cod, herring, salmon, sardines, mackerel and trout is significant. The amount of omega-3s may vary according to the composition of fish that fish consume, growing conditions and locations. Farmed fish may have higher levels of EPA and DHA than wild-caught fish. These considerations may affect flavor and cost.

Wild Atlantic salmon contains about 1.22 grams of DHA and 0.35 grams of EPA per 3-ounce serving. In comparison, sardines contain about 0.74 grams of DHA and 0.45 grams of EPA per 3-ounce serving and wild rainbow trout contains about 0.44 grams of DHA and 0.40 grams of EPA per 3-ounce serving.

FAT DIGESTION, ABSORPTION, METABOLISM AND STORAGE

In general, the more solidified the fat or oil, the more challenging it is for the body to process, use, eliminate or store. Monounsaturated and polyunsaturated fatty acids that are found in avocados, nuts and plant oils are largely easier for the body to handle. Saturated fats that are found in cheese, meats and milk as well as coconuts and palm products are acceptable on a ketogenic diet if consumed in moderation. Their role in cardiovascular disease is still of concern.

Avocados, beef fat, butter, mayonnaise, nut butters, poultry skin and salad dressings have delicious mouth feel due to their unique compositions of fats and oils. From the moment these buttery, creamy and smooth foods are consumed, their complex fat digestion begins.

FAT DIGESTION

Fat digestion begins in the mouth, where it is mostly physical. The teeth tear apart fatty foods and the temperature within the mouth melts some of the fats. A gland under the tongue also secretes a fat-splitting enzyme called lipase.

Then the fatty residue passes through the esophagus into the stomach, where it mixes with gastric lipase, an enzyme that is secreted by the stomach cells. Gastric lipase continues fat digestion as the stomach muscles churn and mix the stomach contents. Together, this process continues to break down the fat by breaking up large fat molecules into smaller ones and evenly distributing them.

Most of the fats in foods and beverages are packaged in the form of triglycerides, which must be broken down into fatty acids and a molecule called glycerol for absorption. This process tends to be slow. As a result, fats tend to linger in the stomach and contribute to fullness or satiety. This can take up to a few hours and is why a fatty meal is so filling and why a low-fat meal may be so unsatisfying. One of the plusses of the ketogenic diet is a lack of hunger.

Most fat digestion happens after fat passes from the stomach to the small intestine. Once the fatty residue moves inside the small intestine, the smallest fatty acids and glycerol are able to pass through the intestinal wall into the blood. They are transported to the liver where they are converted into energy and other fats as needed. Sometimes the liver stores fat, which is not a healthy condition.

The larger triglycerides are broken down in the small intestine by bile, an emulsifier that is made in the liver and stored in the gallbladder. Bile emulsifies fats by breaking them down with watery digestive secretions and prepares them for additional breakdown by enzymes. The pancreas then secretes a digestive enzyme into the small intestine, which breaks down the emulsified triglycerides even further.

FAT ABSORPTION

Fatty acids and cholesterol cannot easily travel in the blood or in the lymph, a watery body fluid that carries the products of fat digestion. This is because they are large molecules, and fat and water do not mix (think oil and vinegar salad dressing that must be shaken before using).

To compensate, fatty acids are packaged inside a protein "shell" for their journey through the bloodstream. These protein packages are called lipoproteins, which means lipids (fats) and protein. The two most well known types of lipoproteins are low-density lipoproteins (LDL) and high-density lipoproteins (HDL), both discussed in regards to cholesterol on pages 8-9.

HDLs contain the most protein and the least fats and carry cholesterol to the liver for recycling or disposal, while LDLs contain mostly cholesterol. This protein to fat ratio is another reason why HDLs are considered to be "good" cholesterol and LDLs "bad" cholesterol for the body.

The fatty acids that are not used by the body are returned to the liver for recycling, disposal or storage. Excess fat in the diet may contribute to greater fat stores. But on a ketogenic diet fat is converted into energy. The majority of body cells can use fatty acids for energy when glucose is not available, except for those in the brain, eyes and red blood cells that rely upon glucose.

When carbohydrates are limited, as in the ketogenic diet, the brain can still obtain a small amount of glucose from a process called gluconeogenesis (glucose production from fats and proteins). On a ketogenic diet, the brain mainly uses ketones for one-half to three-quarters of its energy needs. This process was likely created as a survival mechanism by the body when carbohydrates were limited.

FAT METABOLISM

After dietary fats are digested and absorbed they can be channeled into energy production. Additionally, enzymes can break down stored fats to release fatty acids into the bloodstream. When these fatty acids reach the muscle cells, they go into the powerhouse of the cell, called the mitochondria.

AFTER DIETARY FATS ARE DIGESTED AND ABSORBED THEY CAN BE CHANNELED INTO ENERGY PRODUCTION.

In the mitochondria, energy (calories) is removed from the fatty acids that produce chemical energy for metabolism. Carbon dioxide and water are by-products.

Fats supply about twice the amount of calories for chemical energy production than carbohydrates or protein: 9 calories per gram for fats compared to 4 calories per gram for both carbohydrates and protein. This is why fats and oils are so calorie (and energy) dense.

Another method of fat metabolism or breakdown for energy is called ketosis. Ketosis occurs when there are little to no carbohydrates (the body's preferred energy source) in the diet. Ketosis may occur in prolonged starvation or during higher-protein diets that greatly reduce carbohydrate intake. Ketosis utilizes ketones, the by-products of stored fats, rather than carbohydrates (namely glucose) for energy. *The Ultimate Keto Cookbook* is based on this premise.

FAT STORAGE

Fats that are not used by the body are generally stored in fat cells. Fat cells store small amounts of fat molecules when the concentration of fatty acids in the blood rises, such as after a high-fat meal or snack. An increase in fatty acids in the blood triggers an enzyme called lipase (located in fat tissue) to convert the fatty acids from the blood into a storage form within the fat cells.

The majority of stored fat in the human body is under the skin, called subcutaneous fat. A high percentage of subcutaneous fat surrounds the buttocks, breasts, hips and waist in females—likely for reproduction purposes. In males, most subcutaneous fat is found around the abdomen, buttocks and chest. There is also fat around the kidneys, liver and inside muscles. A goal in a well-designed diet program is to reduce extraneous fat—especially the fat that surrounds the organs and muscles.

METABOLISM: FATS VERSUS CARBOHYDRATES

Since the 1950's, Americans were advised to reduce fat in their diet for heart disease protection, weight loss and weight maintenance and well-being. Dietary approaches were low in fat and cholesterol and higher in carbohydrates (starches and sugars), while higher protein and fat diets were criticized for promoting rich foods and beverages and contributing to elevated blood cholesterol.

During the 1990's when high carbohydrate diets were at their peak in popularity, obesity rates began to rise. Total calories were implicated in these increases, but also the amounts of carbohydrates in the American diet—particularly processed carbohydrates from refined breadstuffs and sugar-filled beverages—were linked with the rise in obesity.

Subsequently, new research demonstrated that low-carbohydrate, higher-fat diets actually improve HDL-cholesterol and do not significantly increase LDL-cholesterol. An examination of carbohydrate metabolism versus fat metabolism explains how this can be possible.

Your body must maintain its blood sugar within a certain range for sufficient energy to think, work, exercise and perform other activities. Insulin, a hormone produced by the pancreas, helps to shift blood sugar (glucose) into the cells for these functions.

Dietary carbohydrates in the form of starches and sugars supply your body with these needed carbohydrates. The body also has a limited store of glycogen or stored carbohydrates—about 2,500 calories—in reserve that are contained within the blood, liver and muscles. However, this amount can quickly be expended to meet the increased energy demands during disease states, exercise and fasting.

In contrast, your body has about 50,000 calories of stored fat with potential energy that it can be converted into energy through a complex series of chemical reactions.

After eating or drinking, insulin moves blood sugar (glucose) into the cells for energy; blood sugar returns to normal levels and you get hungry, eat, and the process repeats. If the pancreas does not produce enough insulin (as in diabetes), this may damage the small blood vessels in the body and blindness, heart attack, infections, kidney disease, stroke or poor wound healing may result. Either oral or injected insulin may be needed—also as in diabetes.

YOUR BODY MUST MAINTAIN ITS BLOOD SUGAR WITHIN A CERTAIN RANGE FOR SUFFICIENT ENERGY TO THINK, WORK, EXERCISE AND PERFORM OTHER ACTIVITIES.

If the body runs out of stored carbohydrates, then the liver produces ketones that can be converted into energy in ketosis (described in Fat Metabolism). A higher-fat lower-carb diet encourages the body to use ketosis for energy production, sparing glucose for the brain, eyes and red blood cells. This shift in energy metabolism generally results in weight loss. Depending upon the degree of ketosis, weight loss may be significant. An in-depth discussion about the ketogenic diet and dieting follows this section.

Carbohydrates contain water, so part of the initial weight loss in a higher protein and fat and lower carbohydrate diet is the decrease in water stores. This is partially the reason why the initial weight loss at the beginning of a ketogenic diet may be significant. Another reason may be that a ketogenic diet differs significantly in food and beverage choices from a standard diet.

There may be some temporary side effects on a ketogenic diet, such as fatigue, light-headedness and/or increased urination. It is important to check first with a healthcare provider before beginning a ketogenic diet—or any diet.

Refined carbohydrates (especially those low in fat) are processed very quickly, and may first spike and then plunge blood sugar levels. Low-fat, refined carbohydrate-containing foods are also quite unsatisfying, which may backfire and cause a person to overeat. Initially the decrease in carbohydrates may be physically and emotionally discomforting, but once the body adjusts to a ketogenic state, more protein and fat in the diet may be satiating. Since fat has twice as many calories per gram as carbohydrates, you may find that you'll actually be more satisfied with less food.

THE KETOGENIC DIET AND DIETING

The ketogenic diet is hardly new. The idea that fasting could be used as a therapy to treat disease was one that ancient Greek and Indian physicians embraced. "On the Sacred Disease", an early treatise in the Hippocratic Corpus, proposed how dietary modifications could be useful in epileptic management. Hippocrates, a Greek physician called the Father of Modern Medicine, wrote in "Epidemics" how abstinence from food and drink cured epilepsy.

In the 20th century, the first ketogenic diet became popularized in the 1920's and 30's as a regimen for treating epilepsy and an alternative to non-mainstream fasting. It was also promoted as a means of restoring health. In 1921, the ketogenic diet was officially established when an endocrinologist noted that three water-soluble compounds were produced by the liver as a result of following a diet that was rich in fat and low in carbohydrates. The term "water diet" had been used prior to this time to describe a diet that was free of starch and sugar. This is because when carbohydrates are broken down by the body carbon dioxide and water are by-products. When newer, anticonvulsant therapies were established, the ketogenic diet was temporarily abandoned.

In the 1960's the ketogenic diet was revisited when it was noted that more ketones are produced by medium chain triglycerides (MCTs) per unit of energy than by normal dietary fats (mostly long-chain triglycerides) because MCTs are quickly transported to the liver to be metabolized. In research diets where about 60 percent of the calories came from MCT oil, more protein and up to about three times as many carbohydrates could be consumed in comparison to "classic" ketogenic diets. This is why MCT oil is included in some ketogenic diets today.

In the 1950's and 1960's many versions of the ketogenic diet were popularized as high-protein, low-carbohydrate and a quick method of weight loss. Also at this time, the risk factors of excess fat and protein in the diet were criticized for being detrimental to health. Outside of the medical community, the ketogenic diet was not widely recognized for its therapeutic benefits so response to it was sensational in scope.

Then in the 1980's the Glycemic Index (GI) of foods and beverages was revealed that accounted for the differences in the speed of digestion of different types of carbohydrates. This explanation became the springboard for a number of ketogenic diets that were revised from years earlier. By the late 1990's the low-carb craze became one of the most popular types of dieting. Since this time, the original ketogenic diet underwent many refinements and hybrid diets developed.

Variations of the ketogenic diet continued to surface throughout the 20th century since the premise of the ketogenic diet—higher fat and protein and low carbohydrate—was used to treat diabetes and induce weight loss among other applications.

TABLE 1

KETOGENIC DIET BASICS

Generally, the percentages of macronutrients on a ketogenic diet are as follows:

- Fat – 60 to 75 percent of total daily calories
- Protein - 15 to 30 percent of total daily calories
- Carbohydrates – 5 to 10 percent of total daily calories

Both fat and protein have high priority on a ketogenic diet, with non-starchy carbohydrates completing the remaining calories. While calories are not as important on the ketogenic diet as they are for other diets, a closer examination of the contributions of these macronutrients helps to put the amounts into perspective.

If total daily calories were about 2,000, then the percentages of macronutrients on a ketogenic diet would resemble the following amounts:

- Fat – 60 to 75 percent of total daily calories or about 1,200 to 1,500 calories
- Protein – 15 to 30 percent of total daily calories or about 300 to 600 calories
- Carbohydrates – 5 to 10 percent of total daily calories or about 100 to 200 calories

In selecting foods and beverages, think protein and fat first, then non-starchy carbohydrates to complete. Until you truly have a handle on what constitutes low carbohydrates, find a carbohydrate counter to help to keep you in line. The ketogenic diet meal suggestions in TABLE 5 – SAMPLE KETOGENIC DIET MEALS: BREAKFASTS, LUNCHES, DINNERS AND SNACKS on page 26 may help your food and beverage selections.

TABLE 2

ADVANTAGES AND DRAWBACKS OF KETOGENIC DIETS

ADVANTAGES	DRAWBACKS
• No calorie counting or focus on portion sizes	• Hard to sustain
• Initial weight loss	• Limited food choices
• After initial transition, hunger subsides	• May lead to taste fatigue
• Improved energy	• Socialization difficult
• Improved blood pressure	• Digestive issues (such as constipation, fatty stool, nausea)
• Improved blood fats: high-density lipoproteins, cholesterol, low-density lipoproteins, triglycerides	• Nutrient deficiencies (such as calcium, vitamins A, C, D, B-vitamins, fiber, magnesium, selenium)
• Reduced blood sugar, C-reactive protein (marker of inflammation), insulin, waist circumference	• Fiber, vitamin and mineral supplements suggested
• Significant short-term weight loss possible	• Increased urination (bladder, kidney contraindications)
	• Diabetes issues
	• Rapid, sizeable short-term weight loss concerning; long-term weight maintenance questionable

Table 1 summarizes the ketogenic diet basics. Many clinical studies examined heir effectiveness and safety and their advantages and drawbacks were identified. These are condensed in **Table 2**.

FAT IN HEALTH AND DISEASE

Fats are essential to the diet and health for many purposes. Fats function as the body's thermostat. The layer of fat just beneath the skin helps to keep the body warm or causes it to perspire to cool the body.

Fat contributes to bile acids, cell membranes and steroid hormones (such as estrogen and testosterone), cushions the body from shock and helps to regulate fluid balance. Too many or too few fats in the diet may influence each of these important body functions.

One of the most important roles of fat in the body is as an energy source, especially when carbohydrates are not available from the diet or are lacking in the body. When people did manual work all day and expended the calories that they consumed, they made good use of carbohydrates and fats in their diet and within their energy stores. Today's laborsaving devices and sedentary lifestyles create less need for excess carbohydrate calories—particularly if they are refined. Even a plant-based diet may be unnecessarily high in refined carbohydrate calories.

Over the years, as humans moved from a plant-based diet toward an animal-based diet, the composition of fatty acids in the American diet switched from monounsaturated and polyunsaturated fats to more saturated fats, which are associated more with cardiovascular disease. A diet that is only filled with saturated fats may not be healthy. By incorporating avocado, fish, nuts, oils and seeds and other foods that contain monounsaturated and polyunsaturated fats into your diet this may help to support a healthier proportion of fats in the body for weight maintenance and good health.

Besides cardiovascular disease, excess saturated and trans fats in the human diet are associated with certain cancers, cerebral vascular disease, diabetes, obesity and metabolic syndrome (a collection of conditions that may include abnormal cholesterol or triglyceride levels, excess body fat around the waist, high blood sugar and increased blood pressure that may increase a person's risk of diabetes, heart disease and/or stroke.

THE CHOLESTEROL CONTROVERSY

Atherosclerosis, or hardening of the arteries, is not a modern disease. Rather, the association between blood cholesterol and cardiovascular disease was recognized as far back as the 1850's.

One hundred years later in the 1950's, cholesterol and saturated fats in the diet were implicated as major risk factors for cardiovascular disease. Then in the 1980's, major US health institutions established that the process of lowering blood cholesterol (specifically LDL-cholesterol) reduces the risk of heart attacks that are caused by coronary heart disease.

Some scientists questioned this conclusion that marked the unofficial start of what's been called the "cholesterol controversy". Studies of cholesterol-lowering drugs known as statins supported the idea that reducing blood cholesterol means less mortality from heart disease. Subsequent statin studies have questioned this association. Other factors aside from dietary cholesterol have since been identified that may lead to elevated blood cholesterol, such as trans fats.

The liver manufactures cholesterol, so reducing cholesterol in the diet should help to reduce blood cholesterol, coronary heart disease and the risk of heart attack. But in some individuals, the liver produces more cholesterol than the body requires and cardiovascular disease may still develop. Accordingly, dietary cholesterol does not necessarily predict cardiovascular disease or a heart attack.

While dietary cholesterol may be a measure for greater cardiovascular risks, cardiovascular disease and heart attacks are also dependent upon such lifestyle and genetic factors as age, diet, exercise, gender, genetics, medication and stress. Reducing hydrogenated fats, saturated fats and trans fats; incorporating mono- and polyunsaturated fats and losing weight to help better manage blood fats are other sensible measures to take.

Longer-term weight management is also a preventative measure in cardiovascular disease. Reducing cholesterol and saturated fat in the diet while integrating foods and beverages with mono- and polyunsaturated fats and oils, dietary fiber, antioxidants and other phytonutrients may lead to a decrease in overall calorie consumption and weight loss and an improvement in overall health.

SO WHAT (AND HOW) SHOULD I EAT?

If you want to lose body fat, then the general consensus is that you need to take in fewer calories than you burn for energy. If you're an average woman over 40, decreasing your caloric intake may be a reasonable starting point. If you are of shorter stature and/or very inactive, or you haven't dropped any pounds after a few weeks at this level, you may consider lowering your daily intake of calories by 100-calorie increments until you start seeing weight loss. But don't go much below 1,000 calories without your health care provider's supervision. (And be sure to check with your health care provider before making any major changes to your diet or activity level, especially if you have any serious health problems.)

Another approach to weight loss is the ketogenic diet that does not focus on calories. Instead, the ketogenic diet focuses on the composition of calories from fats, proteins and carbohydrates.

Fats are satisfying because they take longer for the body to digest, and some are converted into ketones for energy. You don't want to skimp on proteins because protein helps maintain and build calorie-burning muscle and also keeps you satiated between meals. Choose protein sources that supply monounsaturated fats and other heart-healthy unsaturated fats; good options include fish, seafood, nuts and seeds. (Fatty fish, such as herring, mackerel, salmon and tuna contain polyunsaturated fats—especially disease-fighting omega-3 fatty acids). You'll need to replace highly processed and refined foods that are full of saturated and trans fats, sugar and refined carbohydrates with minimally processed fiber- and nutrient-rich foods that include non-starchy vegetables

> WHAT YOU'LL LIKELY END UP WITH IS A SATISFYING EATING PLAN WITH AMPLE PROTEIN, HEALTHY FATS AND MINIMAL CARBOHYDRATES THAT MAY HELP YOU TO FEEL FULL AND LOSE WEIGHT IN THE PROCESS.

What you'll likely end up with is a satisfying eating plan with ample protein, healthy fats and minimal carbohydrates that may help you to feel full and lose weight in the process. It's also a plan that may help you to maintain weight loss over time in a modified manner.

If you've ever tried to lose weight before, you know how quickly between-meal hunger may sabotage your best efforts. When your stomach starts rumbling hours before your next meal, it's tempting to grab whatever is available. Often, that "whatever" is some unhealthy packaged snack food or beverage that is loaded with empty calories, sodium, sugars and/or unhealthy fats. Or, if you manage to ignore this hunger, you may become so ravenous at the next meal that you consume far more calories than your body actually needs.

To prevent hunger from spoiling your weight-loss efforts, eat when you are hungry and stop eating when you are full, whether a meal or snack. Try to consume meals and snacks that include a source of hunger-fighting protein and healthy fat, and count your carbs so as not to exceed the daily limit of 20 to 50 grams of non-starchy carbohydrates.

TABLE 3

ACCEPTABLE FOODS, BEVERAGES AND INGREDIENTS FOR KETOGENIC DIETS

BEVERAGES

- Broth
- Hard liquor
- Nut milks
- Unsweetened coffee, tea
- Water

EGGS

- Egg whites
- Powdered eggs
- Whole eggs

FATS AND OILS

- Butter
- Cocoa butter
- Coconut butter, cream and oil
- Ghee
- Lard
- Oils: avocado oil, macadamia nut oil, MCT oil, olive oil and cold-pressed vegetable oils (flax, safflower, soybean)
- Mayonnaise

FISH AND SEAFOOD

- Anchovies
- Fish (catfish, cod, flounder, halibut, mackerel, mahi-mahi, salmon, snapper, trout, tuna)
- Shellfish (clams, crab, lobster, mussels, oysters, scallops, squid)

FRUITS AND VEGETABLES

- Avocados
- Cruciferous vegetables (broccoli, Brussels sprouts, cabbage, cauliflower, kohlrabi)
- Fermented vegetables (kimchi, saurkraut)
- Leafy greens (bok choy, chard, endive, lettuce, kale, radicchio, spinach, watercress)
- Lemon and lime juice and zest
- Mushrooms
- Non-starchy vegetables (asparagus, bamboo shoots, celery, cucumber
- Seaweed and kelp
- squash (spaghetti squash, yellow squash, zucchini)
- Tomatoes (in some ketogenic diets, tomatoes are used in moderation)

DAIRY PRODUCTS

- Crème fraîche
- Greek yogurt
- Hard cheese (aged Cheddar, feta, Parmesan, Swiss)
- Heavy whipping cream
- Soft cheese (brie, blue, Colby, Monterey Jack, mozzarella)
- Sour cream
- Spreadable cheese (cream cheese, cottage cheese and mascarpone)

MEATS AND POULTRY

- Beef (ground beef, roasts, steak, stew meat)
- Goat (leg, loin, rack, saddle, shoulder)
- Lamb (leg, loin, rack, ribs, shank, shoulder)
- Organ meats (heart, kidneys, liver, tongue)
- Poultry with skin (such as chicken, duck, pheasant, quail, turkey)
- Pork (bacon and sausage without fillers, ground pork, ham, pork chops, pork loin, tenderloin)
- Tofu (in some ketogenic diets, soy products are used in moderation)
- Veal (double, flank, leg, rib, shoulder, sirloin)

NON-DAIRY BEVERAGES

- Almond milk
- Cashew milk
- Coconut milk
- Soymilk (in some ketogenic diets, soy products are used in moderation)

NUTS AND SEEDS

- Nut butters (almond, macadamia)
- Seeds (chia, flax, poppy, sesame, sunflower)
- Whole nuts (almonds, Brazil nuts, macadamia, pecans, hazelnuts, peanuts, pine nuts, walnuts)

PANTRY ITEMS

- Coffee (unsweetened)
- Herbs (dried or fresh such as basil, cilantro, oregano, parsley, rosemary and thyme)
- Horseradish
- Hot sauce
- Mustard
- Pepper
- Pesto sauce
- Pickles
- Salad dressings (without sweeteners)
- Salt
- Spices (such as cayenne pepper, chili powder, cinnamon and cumin)
- Tea (unsweetened)
- Unsweetened gelatin
- Vinegar
- Whey protein (unsweetened)
- Worcestershire sauce

TABLE 4

UNACCEPTABLE FOODS, BEVERAGES AND INGREDIENTS FOR KETOGENIC DIETS

- Alcohol other than hard liquor (beer, sugary alcoholic beverages, wine)
- Beans
- Breads and breadstuffs
- Cakes and pastries
- Candy
- Cereals
- Cookies
- Crackers
- Flours
- Fruit, all (fresh, dried)
- Grains (amaranth, barley, buckwheat, bulgur, corn, millet, oats, rice, rye, sorghum, sprouted grains, wheat)
- Legumes (lentils, peas)
- Margarines with trans fats
- Milk (some full-fat milk is acceptable in some ketogenic diets)
- Oats and muesli
- Potatoes, all kinds (white, yellow, sweet)
- Quinoa
- Pasta
- Pizza
- Processed and refined snack foods
- Rice
- Root vegetables
- Soda
- Sports drinks
- Sugar and honey
- Syrup
- Wheat gluten
- Yams

Drink plenty of water throughout the day (especially if you live in a hot climate or sweat excessively) since ketogenic diets tend to be dehydrating and may lead to fatigue or ill feelings. This may be due to an imbalance of electrolytes; specifically sodium that the kidneys excrete during ketosis. Sometimes lightly salting your food may help to restore sodium. A high quality vitamin and mineral supplement is also sensible.

NOTES ON KETOGENIC FOODS, BEVERAGES AND INGREDIENTS

In general, the foods, beverages and ingredients that are included in a ketogenic diet incorporate eggs, healthy fats and oils, fish, meats and organ meats and non-starchy vegetables. These "acceptable" foods, beverages and ingredients contain protein and fats and are low in carbohydrates that contribute to the effectiveness of ketogenic diets. They are listed in **TABLE 3 – ACCEPTABLE FOODS, BEVERAGES AND INGREDIENTS FOR KETOGENIC DIETS**.

In **TABLE 4 – UNACCEPTABLE FOODS, BEVERAGES AND INGREDIENTS FOR KETOGENIC DIETS** are shown. While there is a wide-range of ketogenic diet approaches, these foods, beverages and ingredients are generally considered to be "unacceptable" on many ketogenic diets. In general, their carbohydrate content exceeds what is considered as optimal for effective ketosis and diet success.

TABLE 5

SAMPLE KETOGENIC DIET MEALS: BREAKFAST, LUNCH, DINNER AND SNACKS

Examples of combinations of protein, low-carb, non-starchy vegetables and fats:

BREAKFAST:

- Almond, coconut, hemp or other nut or seed milks or beverages (unsweetened)
- Bacon, sausage or sliced meats (without carbohydrate fillers)
- Cheese, hard or soft varieties
- Eggs with low-carb vegetables (asparagus, broccoli, garlic, mushrooms, onions or spinach) with coconut or olive oil, topped with avocado, olives, salsa and/ or sour cream
- Greek yogurt with nut butter, chia or flax seeds, herbs and spices (cinnamon, ginger or nutmeg)
- Smoked fish (such as lox, sable or whitefish)
- Smoothies made with keto-friendly ingredients (protein powder, almond or coconut butter, avocado, cocoa powder, chia or flax seeds, spices such as cinnamon, smoked paprika or turmeric and unsweetened almond or hemp milk)
- Vegetable slices (cucumber or zucchini or lettuce) topped with cheese

LUNCH AND DINNER:

- Eggs + watercress or spinach + avocado dressing
- Lamb + kale + sesame oil
- Pork + cauliflower + coconut butter
- Poultry + zucchini and yellow squash + extra virgin olive oil
- Salmon + broccoli + mustard sauce
- Sardines + cucumbers and onions + sour cream dressing
- Seafood + leafy green salad + oil and vinegar dressing
- Steak + asparagus + butter sauce
- Tofu + mushrooms and bok choy + ghee
- Tuna + celery + mayonnaise

SNACKS:

- Asparagus with goat cheese dip
- Avocado filled hard-cooked eggs
- Celery stuffed with nut or seed butter
- Cheese and olives on skewers
- Chia and flax seed crackers with cream cheese
- Cucumber and cream cheese spread
- Cream cheese and bacon stuffed celery
- Deviled eggs with fresh herbs and chives
- Greek yogurt with chopped cucumbers
- Guacamole with onions and garlic
- Ham and cheddar or Swiss cheese roll ups
- Mixed nut-coated cheese balls
- Nut butters (such as almond) blended with ricotta cheese
- Olives stuffed with bleu cheese
- Parmesan cheese crisps
- Seeds and seed butters as tahini
- Sliced jicama with herbed cream cheese
- Seaweed wrapped firm tofu

NOTES ON RECIPES

Since whole eggs are no longer considered problematic with regard to cholesterol, they are used freely throughout the recipes, particularly for breakfast in **Chapter 1**, where you'll find low-carb recipes for a Ham and Vegetable Omelet and a Spinach, Pepper and Olive Omelet.

You can snack on a higher protein and fat snacks on a ketogenic diet. Check out Fast Guacamole, Kale Chips, Mini Marinated Beef Skewers and Veggie Packed Pizza in **Chapter 2** for tasty low carb options.

The salads in **Chapter 3** feature Crab Cobb Salad and Tomato, Avocado and Cucumber Salad as starters or entrée salads that are low in carbs but high in taste and satisfaction.

Soups in **Chapter 4** range from Chilled Cucumber Soup to hearty Cioppino, with ample protein and great taste—yet skimpy in carbohydrates.

The meat and poultry recipes in **Chapter 5** showcase a variety of protein options that include robust Chili Roasted Turkey with Cilantro-Lime Butternut Squash and mouth-watering Skirt Steak with Red Pepper Chimichurri.

Fish and seafood dishes in **Chapter 6** feature meaty Pan-Seared Halibut Steaks with Avocado Salsa and tasty Trout Stuffed with Fresh Mint and Orange.

You'll discover delicious side dishes in **Chapter 7** that include Grilled Sesame Asparagus and Mashed Cauliflower that are big on taste and light on carbs.

The recipes in this book show that food filled with fats and proteins and non-starchy carbohydrates may be delicious and fit into a ketogenic diet regimen. You can lose and maintain weight by consuming fats and proteins with non-starchy carbs in the right proportions. Like any diet, make sure that you discuss the pros and cons with your health care provider to ensure its safety and effectiveness.

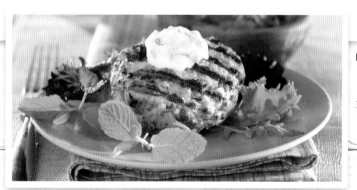

p. 176

BREAKFAST

Vegetable Frittata

MAKES 2 SERVINGS

1 teaspoon canola oil

¼ cup chopped onion

1 clove garlic, minced

¾ cup chopped fresh broccoli

¼ cup chopped fresh mushrooms

½ cup chopped fresh spinach

4 egg whites

⅛ teaspoon salt

Black pepper

2 tablespoons shredded Cheddar, Parmesan or Monterey Jack cheese

1 Preheat broiler. Heat oil in small nonstick ovenproof skillet over medium-high heat. Add onion and garlic; cook and stir 1 minute. Reduce heat to medium. Stir in broccoli and mushrooms; cover and cook over medium heat until broccoli is crisp-tender. Stir in spinach.

2 Meanwhile, whisk egg whites, salt and pepper in small bowl until well blended.

3 Pour egg whites over vegetables in skillet; cook until egg whites are firm but top is still slightly undercooked. Sprinkle with cheese; broil about 2 minutes or until egg whites are cooked through and cheese is melted.

NUTRIENTS PER SERVING

CALORIES
108

TOTAL FAT
5g

SATURATED FAT
2g

CHOLESTEROL
7mg

SODIUM
322mg

CARBOHYDRATE
6g

DIETARY FIBER
1g

PROTEIN
11g

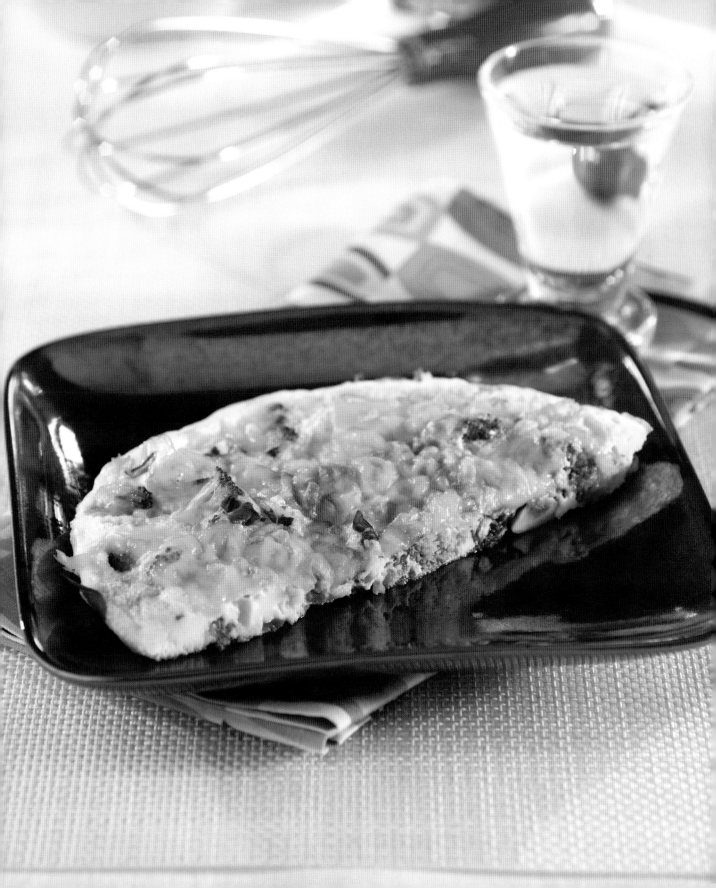

California Omelet with Avocado

MAKES 4 SERVINGS

NUTRIENTS PER SERVING

CALORIES
145

TOTAL FAT
5g

SATURATED FAT
1g

CHOLESTEROL
1mg

SODIUM
389mg

CARBOHYDRATE
13g

DIETARY FIBER
4g

PROTEIN
14g

6 ounces plum tomato, chopped (about 1½ tomatoes)

2 to 4 tablespoons chopped fresh cilantro

¼ teaspoon salt

2 cups cholesterol-free egg substitute *or* 8 eggs

¼ cup milk

1 medium avocado, diced

1 small cucumber, chopped

1 Preheat oven to 200°F. Combine tomatoes, cilantro and salt in small bowl; set aside.

2 Whisk egg substitute and milk in medium bowl until well blended.

3 Heat small nonstick skillet over medium heat; spray with nonstick cooking spray. Pour half of egg mixture into skillet; cook 2 minutes or until eggs begin to set. Lift edge of omelet to allow uncooked portion to flow underneath. Cook 3 minutes or until set.

4 Spoon half of tomato mixture over half of omelet. Loosen omelet with spatula and fold in half. Slide omelet onto serving plates and keep warm in oven. Repeat with remaining egg mixture and tomatoes. Top with avocado and cucumber.

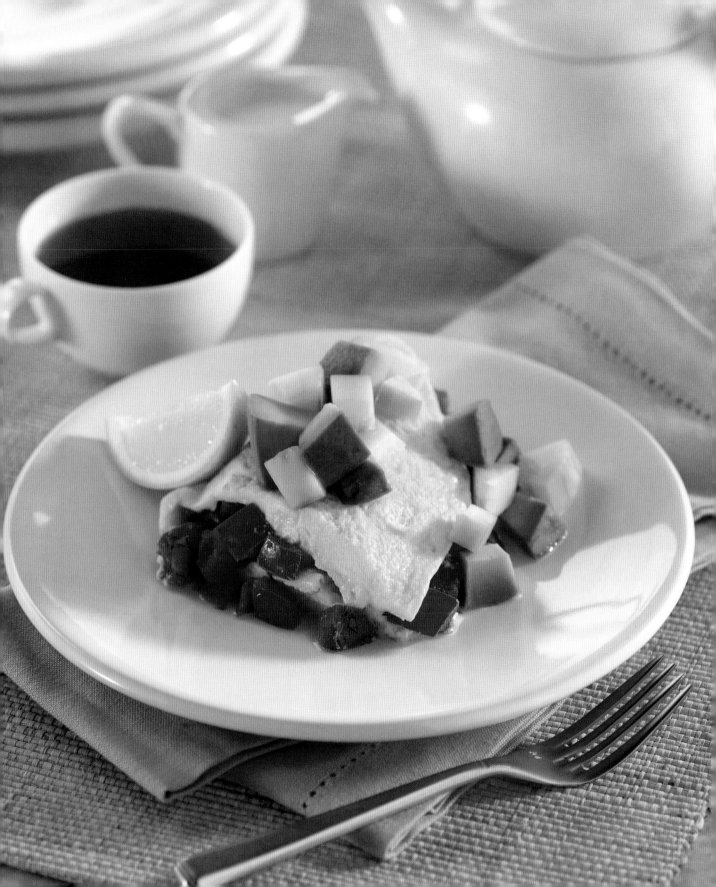

Fabulous Feta Frittata

MAKES 4 SERVINGS

- 8 eggs
- ¼ cup chopped fresh basil
- ¼ cup whipping cream or half-and-half
- ¼ teaspoon salt
- ¼ teaspoon black pepper
- 2 tablespoons butter or olive oil
- 1 package (4 ounces) crumbled feta cheese with basil, olives and sun-dried tomatoes *or* 1 cup crumbled feta cheese
- ¼ cup pine nuts

1 Preheat broiler.

2 Beat eggs, basil, cream, salt and pepper in medium bowl. Melt butter in large ovenproof skillet over medium heat, tilting skillet to coat bottom and side.

3 Pour egg mixture into skillet. Cover and cook 8 to 10 minutes or until eggs are set around edge (center will be wet).

4 Sprinkle cheese and pine nuts evenly over top. Transfer to broiler; broil 4 to 5 inches from heat source 2 minutes or until center is set and pine nuts are golden brown. Cut into wedges to serve.

TIP

If your skillet is not ovenproof, wrap the handle in heavy-duty foil.

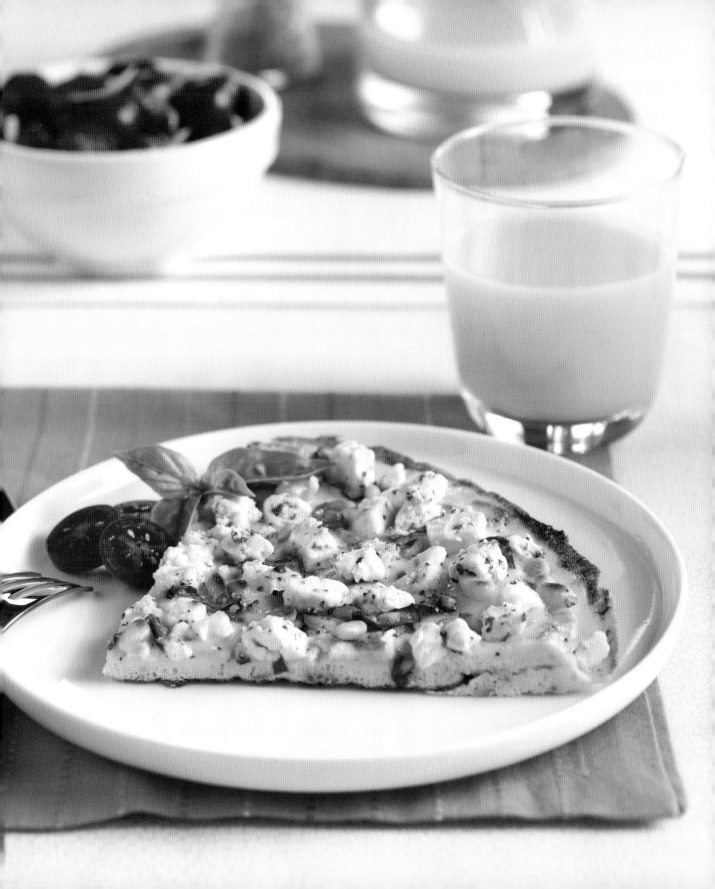

Zucchini Omelet with Dill

MAKES 2 SERVINGS

NUTRIENTS PER SERVING

CALORIES
100

TOTAL FAT
5g

SATURATED FAT
2g

CHOLESTEROL
111mg

SODIUM
290mg

CARBOHYDRATE
3g

DIETARY FIBER
1g

PROTEIN
12g

1 egg
4 egg whites *or* 4 whole eggs
2 tablespoons milk
½ teaspoon dried dill weed
⅛ teaspoon kosher salt
⅛ teaspoon black pepper
1 teaspoon butter
1 cup diced zucchini

1 Whisk egg, egg whites, milk, dill, salt and pepper in medium bowl until blended.

2 Spray medium skillet with nonstick cooking spray. Add butter; cook over medium-high heat until butter is melted. Add zucchini; cook and stir 4 minutes or until lightly browned.

3 Add egg mixture; cook 2 minutes or until eggs begin to set. Lift edge of omelet to allow uncooked portion to flow underneath. Cook 3 minutes or until set. Fold omelet over and cut in half.

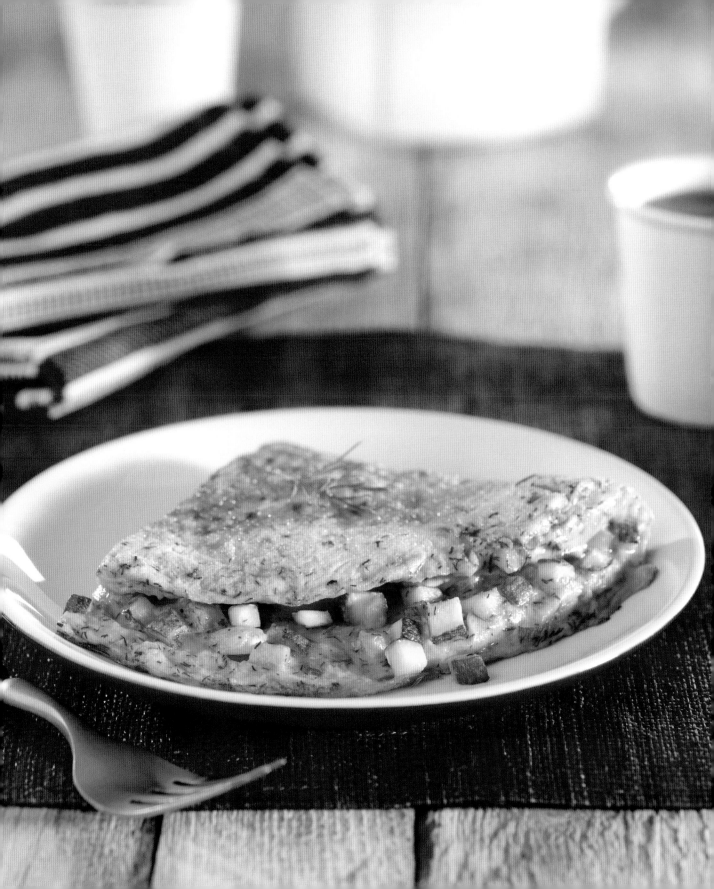

Spinach, Pepper and Olive Omelet

MAKES 4 SERVINGS

NUTRIENTS PER SERVING

CALORIES
152

TOTAL FAT
7g

SATURATED FAT
3g

CHOLESTEROL
11mg

SODIUM
536mg

CARBOHYDRATE
7g

DIETARY FIBER
2g

PROTEIN
16g

1 cup diced red bell pepper

½ teaspoon dried rosemary

⅛ teaspoon red pepper flakes

2 cups loosely packed baby spinach (2 ounces), coarsely chopped

16 stuffed green olives, such as manzanilla, sliced

2 tablespoons chopped fresh basil

2 cups cholesterol-free egg substitute *or* 8 eggs

3 tablespoons milk

2 ounces crumbled goat cheese or reduced-fat feta cheese, divided

1 Spray medium skillet with nonstick cooking spray; heat over medium-high heat. Add bell pepper, rosemary and red pepper flakes; cook and stir 4 minutes or until soft. Remove from heat; stir in spinach, olives and basil. Place in medium bowl; cover and let stand to wilt spinach.

2 Whisk egg substitute and milk in another medium bowl until well blended. Wipe out skillet with paper towel. Spray skillet with cooking spray; heat over medium heat. Add half of egg mixture; cook 2 minutes or until eggs begin to set. Lift edge of omelet to allow uncooked portion to flow underneath. Cook 3 minutes or until set.

3 Top with half of spinach mixture and half of cheese. Loosen omelet with spatula and fold in half. Slide omelet onto serving plate and cover with foil to keep warm. Repeat with remaining ingredients.

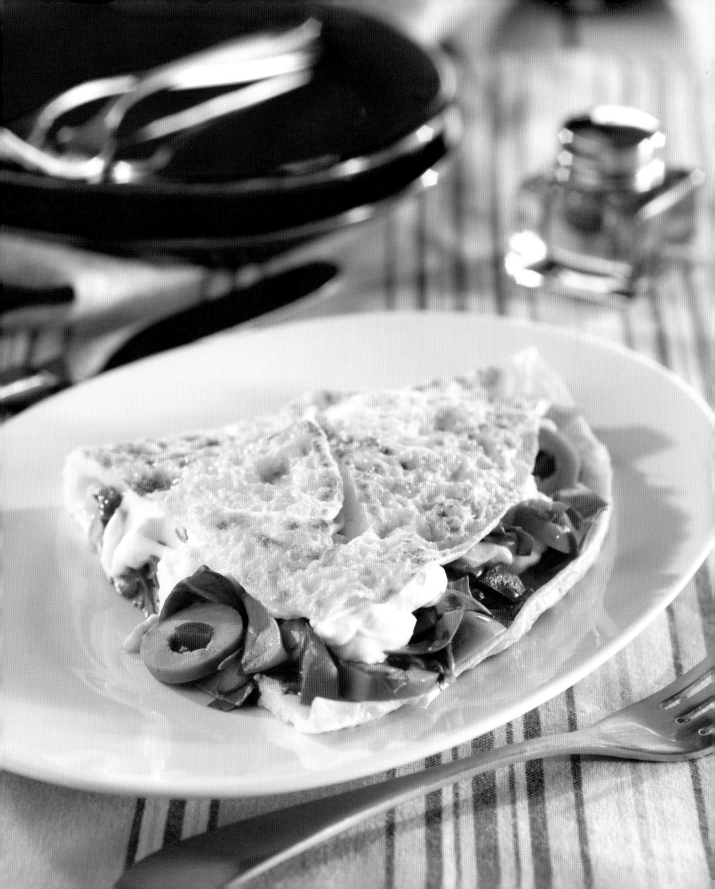

Feta Brunch Bake

MAKES 4 SERVINGS

1 medium red bell pepper

2 bags (10 ounces each) fresh spinach*

6 eggs

1½ cups (6 ounces) crumbled feta cheese

⅓ cup chopped onion

2 tablespoons chopped fresh parsley

¼ teaspoon dried dill weed

Salt and black pepper

Or use 2 packages (10 ounces each) frozen chopped spinach, thawed and squeezed dry. Skip step 2 and add spinach to egg mixture in step 4.

1 Preheat broiler. Place bell pepper on foil-lined broiler pan. Broil 4 inches from heat source 15 to 20 minutes or until blackened on all sides, turning every 5 minutes with tongs. Place in paper bag; close bag and set aside to cool 15 to 20 minutes. Cut around core, twist and remove. Cut bell pepper in half and rub off skin; rinse under cold water. Cut into ½-inch pieces.

2 Fill medium saucepan half full with water; bring to a boil over high heat. Add spinach. Return to a boil; boil 2 to 3 minutes or until wilted. Drain; immediately plunge spinach into medium bowl of cold water. Drain; let stand until cool enough to handle. Squeeze spinach to remove excess water; finely chop.

3 Preheat oven to 400°F. Grease 1-quart baking dish.

4 Whisk eggs in large bowl until foamy. Stir in bell pepper, spinach, cheese, onion, parsley, dill weed and black pepper. Pour egg mixture into prepared dish.

5 Bake 20 minutes or until set. Let stand 5 minutes before serving.

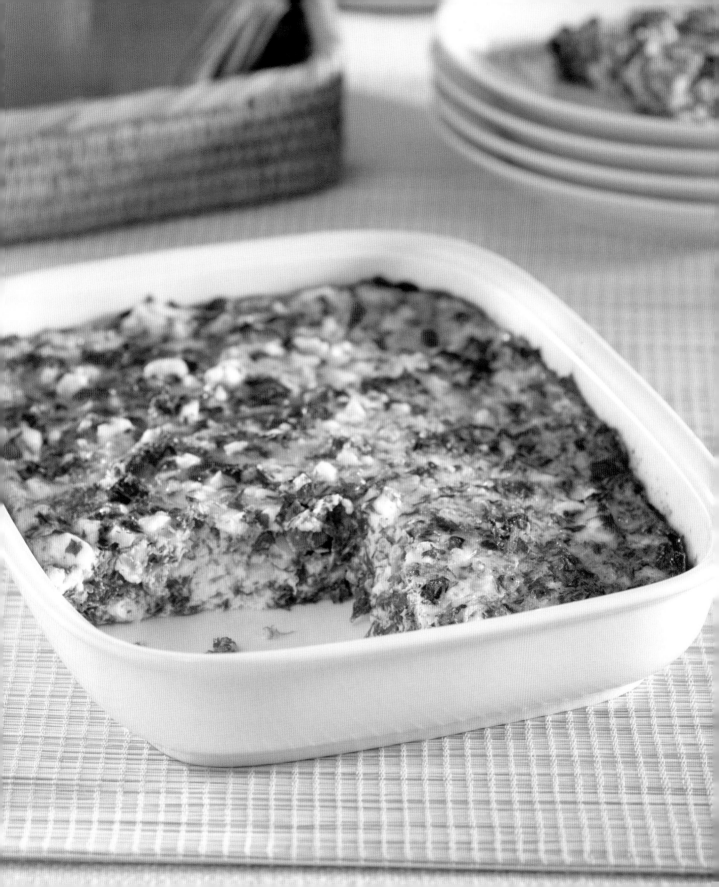

Joe's Special

MAKES 4 TO 6 SERVINGS

Nonstick cooking spray *or* 2 teaspoons olive oil

1 pound lean ground beef

2 cups sliced mushrooms

1 small chopped onion

2 teaspoons Worcestershire sauce

1 teaspoon dried oregano

1 teaspoon ground nutmeg

½ teaspoon garlic powder

½ teaspoon salt

1 package (10 ounces) frozen chopped spinach, thawed

4 eggs, lightly beaten

⅓ cup grated Parmesan cheese

1 Spray large skillet with cooking spray or place oil in skillet; heat over medium-high heat. Add ground beef, mushrooms and onion; cook and stir 6 to 8 minutes or until meat is browned. Add Worcestershire sauce, oregano, nutmeg, garlic powder and salt.

2 Drain spinach (do not squeeze dry); stir into meat mixture. Push mixture to one side of pan. Reduce heat to medium. Pour eggs into other side of pan; cook without stirring 1 to 2 minutes or until set on bottom. Lift eggs to allow uncooked portion to flow underneath. Repeat until softly set. Gently stir into meat mixture and heat through. Stir in cheese.

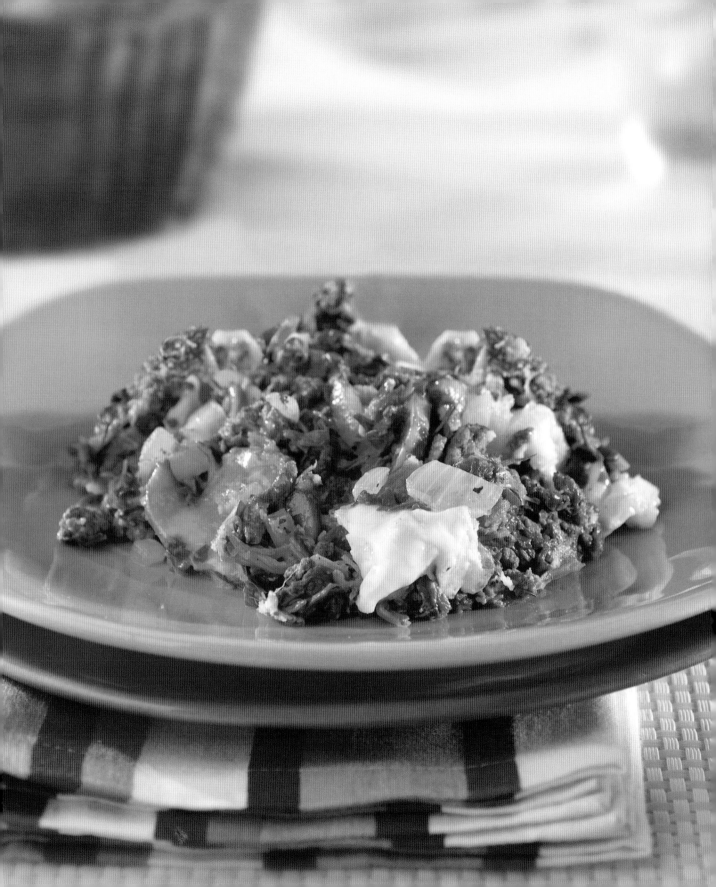

Ham and Vegetable Omelet

MAKES 4 SERVINGS

NUTRIENTS
PER SERVING

CALORIES
126

TOTAL FAT
4g

SATURATED FAT
2g

CHOLESTEROL
17mg

SODIUM
443mg

CARBOHYDRATE
8g

DIETARY FIBER
1g

PROTEIN
16g

Nonstick cooking spray *or* 2 teaspoons olive oil

2 ounces (about ½ cup) diced ham

1 small onion, diced

½ medium green bell pepper, diced

½ medium red bell pepper, diced

2 cloves garlic, minced

1½ cups cholesterol-free egg substitute *or* 6 eggs, lightly beaten

⅛ teaspoon black pepper

½ cup (2 ounces) shredded reduced-fat Colby cheese, divided

1 medium tomato, chopped

1 Spray large skillet with cooking spray or place oil in skillet; heat over medium-high heat. Add ham, onion, bell peppers and garlic; cook and stir 5 minutes or until vegetables are crisp-tender. Transfer mixture to large bowl.

2 Wipe out skillet with paper towel; spray with cooking spray. Heat over medium-high heat. Pour egg substitute into skillet; sprinkle with black pepper. Cook 2 minutes or until bottom is set, lifting edge of egg with spatula to allow uncooked portion to flow underneath. Reduce heat to medium-low; cover and cook 4 minutes or until top is set.

3 Gently slide omelet onto large serving plate; spoon ham mixture down center. Sprinkle with ¼ cup cheese. Carefully fold two sides of omelet over ham mixture; sprinkle with remaining ¼ cup cheese and tomato. Cut into 4 pieces; serve immediately.

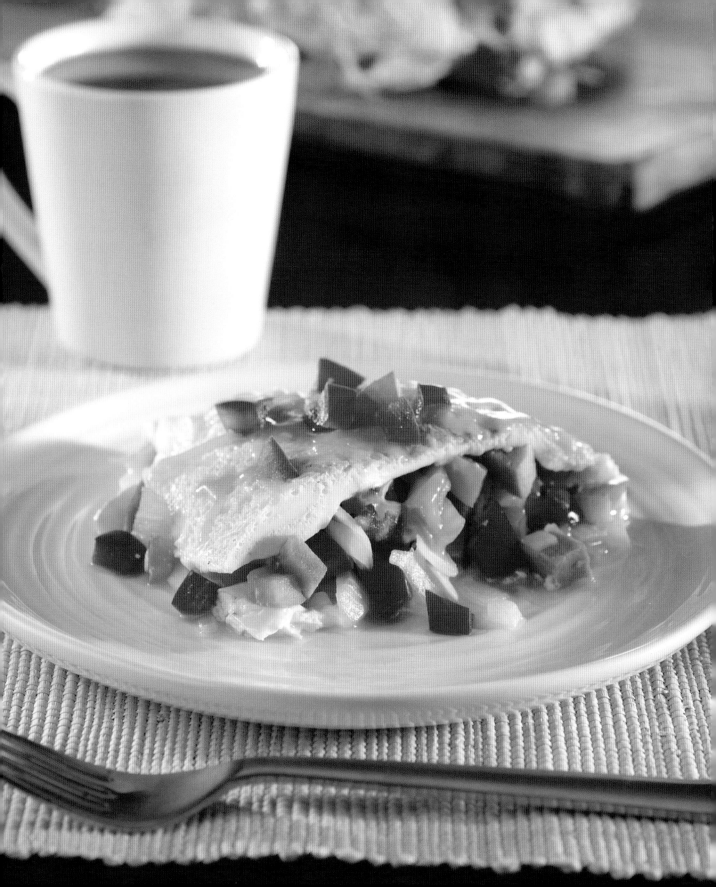

Sausage and Cheddar Omelet

MAKES 4 SERVINGS

NUTRIENTS PER SERVING	
CALORIES	133
TOTAL FAT	6g
SATURATED FAT	3g
CHOLESTEROL	19mg
SODIUM	523mg
CARBOHYDRATE	4g
DIETARY FIBER	1g
PROTEIN	15g

2 uncooked turkey breakfast sausage links (about 1 ounce each)

1 small onion, diced

Nonstick cooking spray *or* 2 teaspoons olive oil

1½ cups cholesterol-free egg substitute *or* 6 eggs, lightly beaten

⅛ teaspoon salt

¼ teaspoon black pepper

½ cup (2 ounces) shredded reduced-fat Cheddar cheese, divided

Sliced green onions (optional)

1 Heat 12-inch nonstick skillet over medium-high heat. Remove sausage from casings. Add sausage and diced onion to skillet. Cook about 5 minutes or until sausage is no longer pink and onion is crisp-tender, stirring to break up meat. Transfer to bowl.

2 Wipe out skillet with paper towel; spray with cooking spray or place oil in skillet. Heat over medium-high heat. Pour egg substitute into skillet; sprinkle with salt and pepper. Cook 2 minutes or until bottom is set, lifting edge of egg to allow uncooked portion to flow underneath. Reduce heat to medium-low. Cover; cook 4 minutes or until top is set.

3 Gently slide cooked egg onto large serving plate; spoon sausage mixture down center. Sprinkle with ¼ cup cheese. Fold sides of omelet over sausage mixture. Sprinkle with remaining ¼ cup cheese and green onions, if desired. Cut into 4 pieces; serve immediately.

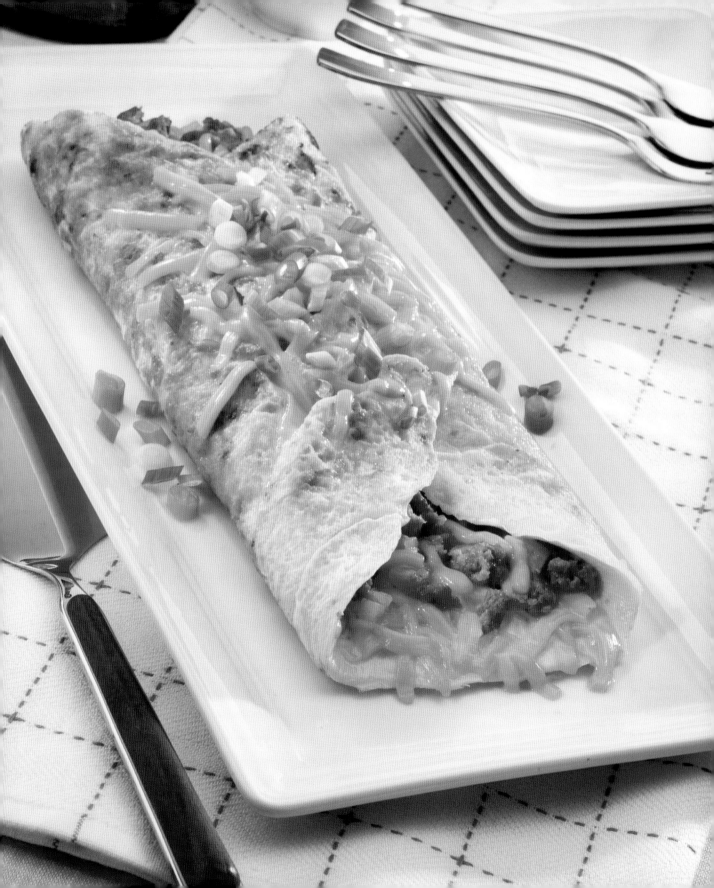

Goat Cheese and Tomato Omelet

MAKES 2 SERVINGS

3 egg whites*

2 eggs*

1 tablespoon water

⅛ teaspoon salt

⅛ teaspoon black pepper

Nonstick cooking spray *or* 2 teaspoons olive oil

⅓ cup crumbled goat cheese

1 medium plum tomato, diced

2 tablespoons chopped fresh basil or parsley

Or use 5 whole eggs.

1 Whisk together egg whites, eggs, water, salt and pepper in medium bowl.

2 Spray medium nonstick skillet with cooking spray or place oil in skillet; heat over medium heat. Add egg mixture; cook 2 minutes or until eggs begin to set on bottom. Lift edge of omelet to allow uncooked portion of eggs to flow underneath. Cook 3 minutes or until center is almost set.

3 Sprinkle cheese, tomato and basil in center of omelet. Fold omelet in half over filling. Cook 1 to 2 minutes or until cheese begins to melt and center is set. Cut omelet in half; transfer to serving plates.

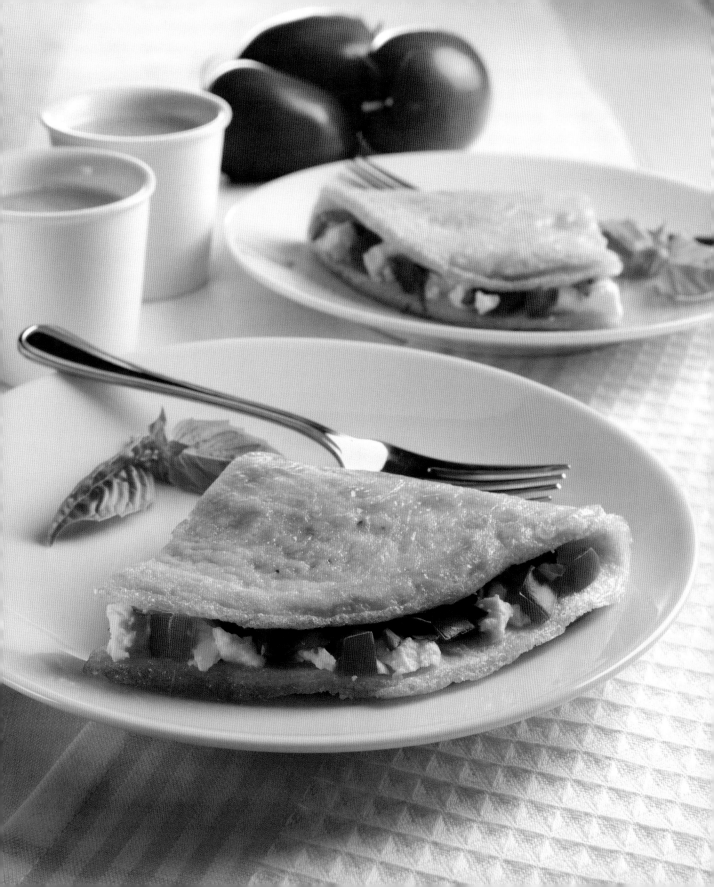

Scrambled Egg and Zucchini Pie

MAKES 2 SERVINGS

NUTRIENTS PER SERVING

CALORIES
140

TOTAL FAT
11g

SATURATED FAT
5g

CHOLESTEROL
235mg

SODIUM
530mg

CARBOHYDRATE
3g

DIETARY FIBER
1g

PROTEIN
11g

2 eggs
2 tablespoons grated Parmesan or Cheddar cheese

¼ teaspoon salt
2 teaspoons butter
1 small zucchini, diced

1 Preheat oven to 350°F.

2 Whisk eggs in small bowl; stir in cheese and salt.

3 Melt butter in small nonstick ovenproof skillet over medium-high heat. Add zucchini; cook and stir 2 to 3 minutes or until crisp-tender. Reduce heat to low; add egg mixture. Cook without stirring 4 to 5 minutes or until eggs begin to set around edge.

4 Transfer skillet to oven and bake 5 minutes or until eggs are set. Cut into wedges to serve.

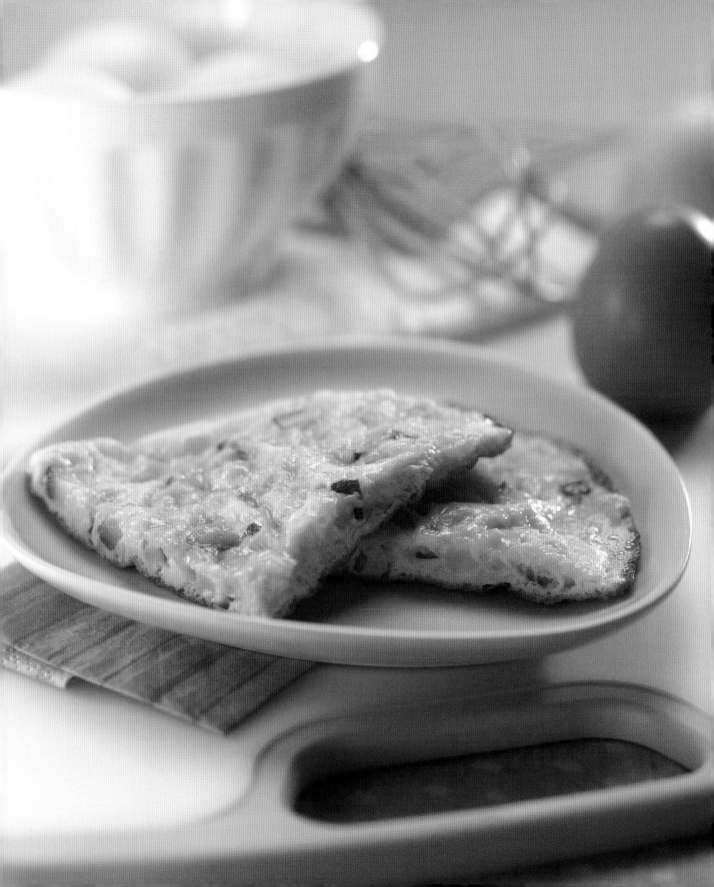

SNACKS

Prosciutto-Wrapped Asparagus with Garlic Mayonnaise

MAKES 8 SERVINGS

2 tablespoons olive oil, divided	Black pepper (optional)
1 package (about 3 ounces) prosciutto, cut lengthwise into 16 strips	¾ cup mayonnaise
	1 teaspoon lemon juice
16 medium asparagus spears, trimmed	1 clove garlic, minced

1 Preheat oven to 400°F. Brush large baking sheet with 1 tablespoon oil. Wrap 1 piece of prosciutto around each asparagus spear. Place asparagus on prepared baking sheet. Brush asparagus with remaining oil; sprinkle with pepper, if desired.

2 Bake about 12 minutes or until asparagus is tender. Cool slightly.

3 Meanwhile for garlic mayonnaise, combine mayonnaise, lemon juice and garlic in small bowl until well blended. Serve asparagus warm with garlic mayonnaise.

NUTRIENTS PER SERVING

CALORIES	210
TOTAL FAT	20g
SATURATED FAT	4g
CHOLESTEROL	20mg
SODIUM	510mg
CARBOHYDRATE	2g
DIETARY FIBER	1g
PROTEIN	5g

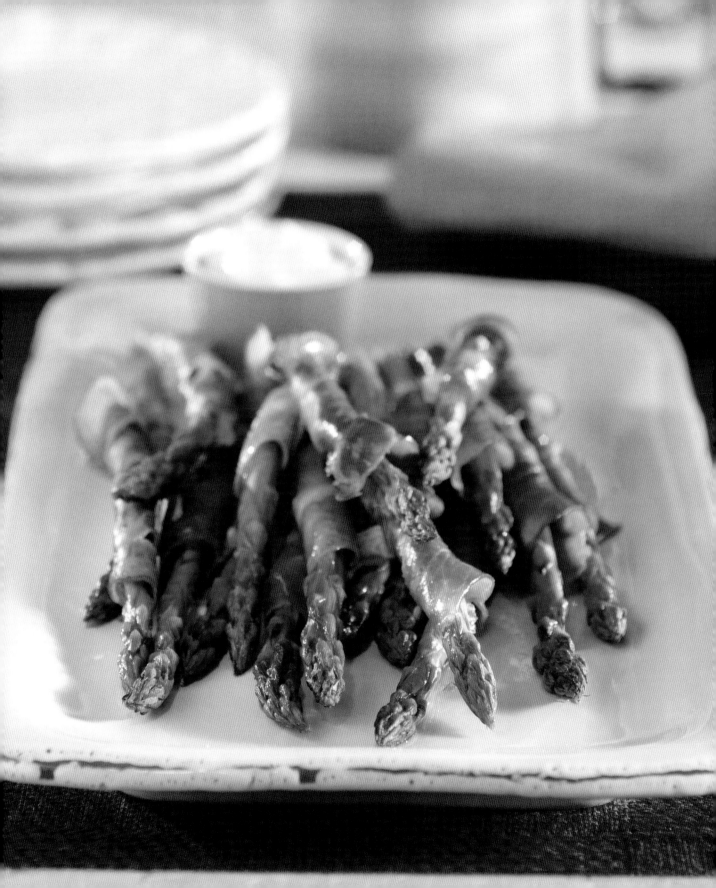

Marinated Antipasto

MAKES 12 APPETIZER SERVINGS (½ CUP PER SERVING)

NUTRIENTS
PER SERVING

CALORIES
130

TOTAL FAT
11g

SATURATED FAT
4g

CHOLESTEROL
5mg

SODIUM
210mg

CARBOHYDRATE
6g

DIETARY FIBER
3g

PROTEIN
5g

¼ cup extra virgin olive oil

2 tablespoons balsamic vinegar

1 clove garlic, minced

½ teaspoon salt

¼ teaspoon black pepper

1 pint (2 cups) cherry tomatoes

1 can (about 14 ounces) quartered artichoke hearts, drained

8 ounces small balls or cubes of fresh mozzarella cheese

1 cup drained pitted kalamata olives

¼ cup sliced fresh basil leaves

Lettuce leaves

1 Whisk oil, vinegar, garlic, salt and pepper in medium bowl. Add tomatoes, artichokes, cheese, olives and basil; toss to coat. Let stand at room temperature 30 minutes.

2 Line platter with lettuce. Arrange antipasto over lettuce; serve at room temperature.

MEAL IDEA

Serve this antipasto as a topping for grilled meat, or add baby spinach or chopped lettuce to make a side dish.

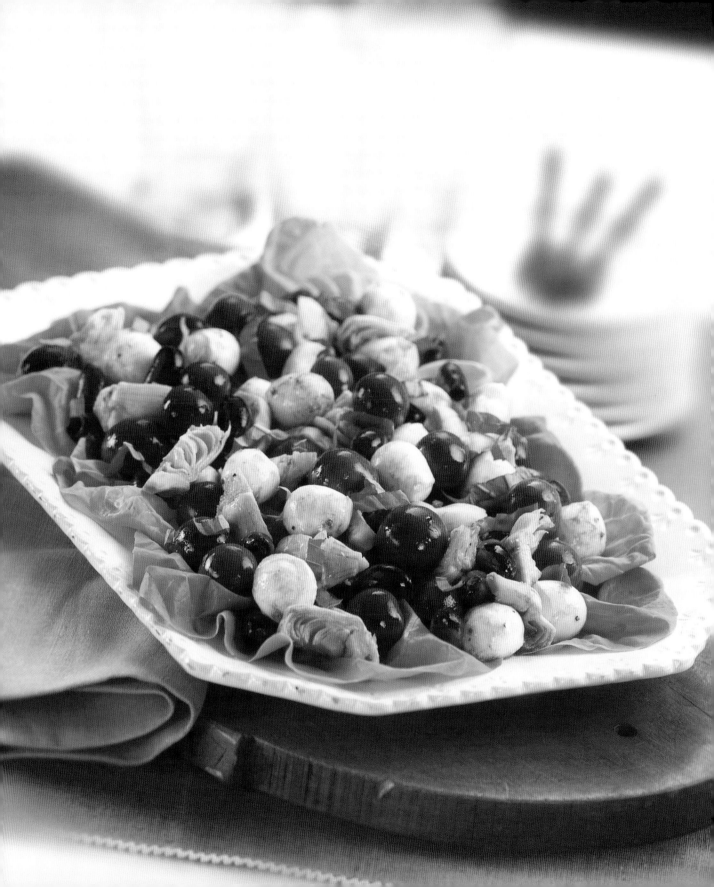

**NUTRIENTS
PER SERVING**

CALORIES
99

TOTAL FAT
7g

SATURATED FAT
3g

CHOLESTEROL
29mg

SODIUM
295mg

CARBOHYDRATE
3g

DIETARY FIBER
1g

PROTEIN
6g

Spinach, Crab and Artichoke Dip

MAKES 10 (¼-CUP) SERVINGS

1 can (6½ ounces) crabmeat, drained and shredded

1 package (10 ounces) frozen chopped spinach, thawed and squeezed dry

1 package (8 ounces) reduced-fat or regular cream cheese

1 jar (about 6 ounces) marinated artichoke hearts, drained and finely chopped

¼ teaspoon hot pepper sauce

Sliced bell peppers and cucumbers

SLOW COOKER DIRECTIONS

1 Pick out and discard any shell or cartilage from crabmeat.

2 Combine crabmeat, spinach, cream cheese, artichokes and hot pepper sauce in 1½-quart slow cooker. Cover; cook on HIGH 1½ to 2 hours or until heated through, stirring after 1 hour. Serve with vegetables.

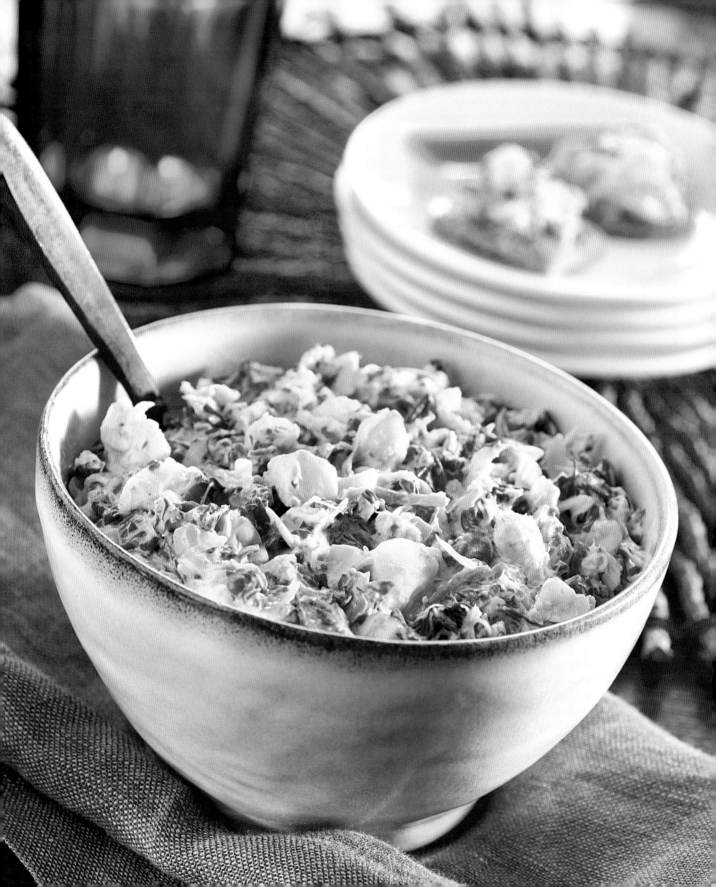

Fast Guacamole

MAKES 8 SERVINGS

2 ripe avocados

½ cup chunky salsa

¼ teaspoon hot pepper sauce (optional)

½ seedless cucumber, sliced into ⅛-inch-thick rounds

1 Cut avocados in half; remove and discard pits. Scoop flesh into medium bowl; mash with fork. Add salsa and hot pepper sauce, if desired; mix well.

2 Transfer guacamole to serving bowl. Serve with cucumber slices.

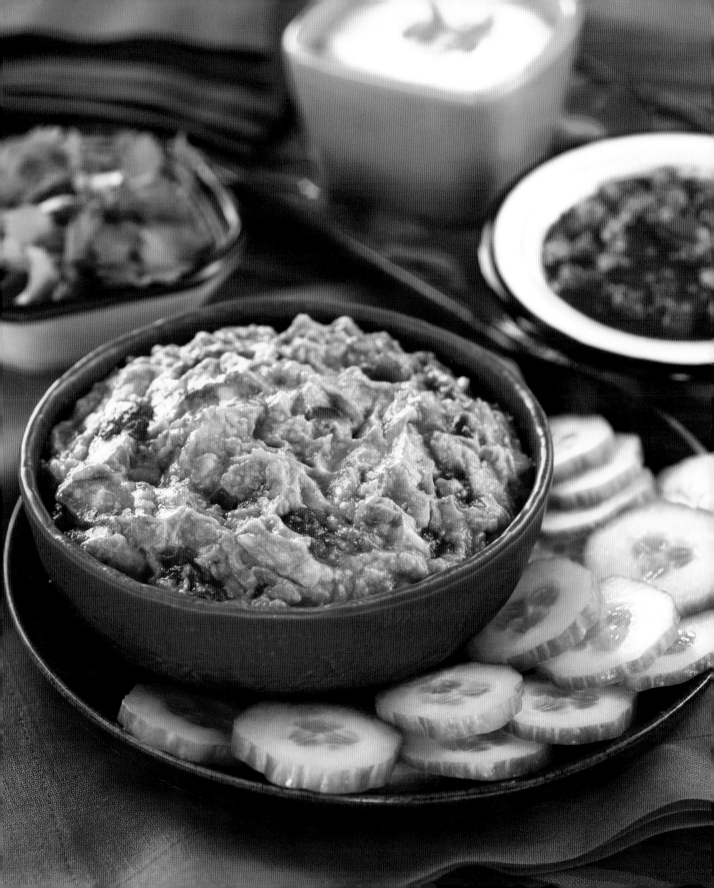

Citrus-Marinated Olives

MAKES 8 SERVINGS (¼ CUP PER SERVING)

NUTRIENTS
PER SERVING

CALORIES
54

TOTAL FAT
6g

SATURATED FAT
0g

CHOLESTEROL
0mg

SODIUM
410mg

CARBOHYDRATE
2g

DIETARY FIBER
2g

PROTEIN
0g

⅓ cup extra virgin olive oil

¼ cup orange juice

3 tablespoons sherry vinegar or red wine vinegar

2 tablespoons lemon juice

1 tablespoon grated orange peel

1 tablespoon grated lemon peel

½ teaspoon ground cumin

¼ teaspoon red pepper flakes

1 cup (about 8 ounces) large green olives, drained

1 cup kalamata olives, rinsed and drained

1 Whisk oil, orange juice, vinegar, lemon juice, orange peel, lemon peel, cumin and red pepper flakes in medium glass bowl. Stir in olives.

2 Let stand overnight at room temperature; refrigerate for up to 2 weeks.

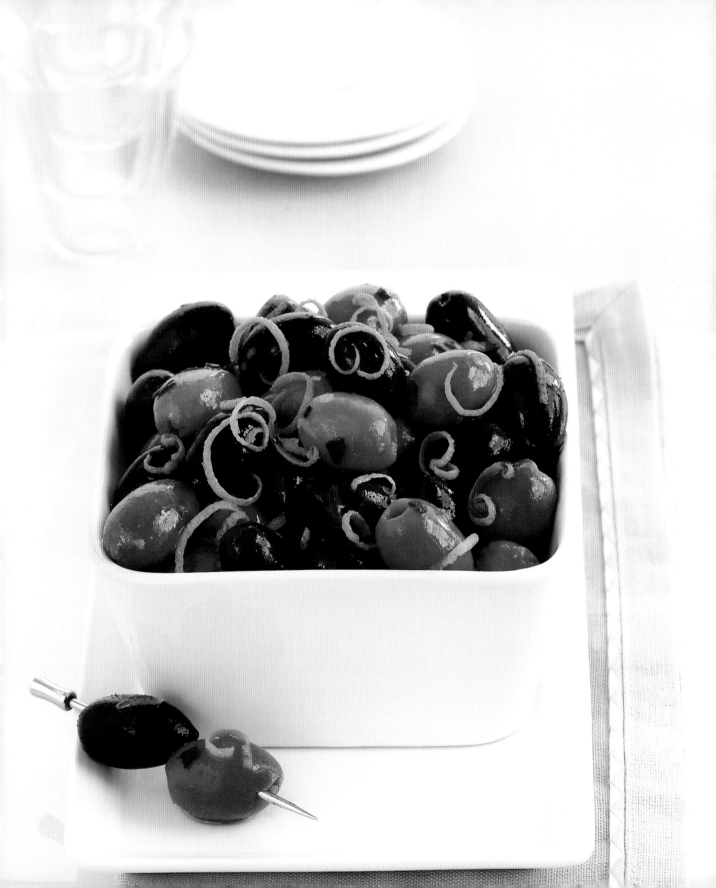

Crispy Cheese Chips

MAKES 8 SERVINGS

1½ cups (6 ounces) shredded mozzarella cheese*

½ cup grated Parmesan cheese

4 green onions

1 teaspoon chili powder

1 teaspoon black pepper

Nonstick cooking spray

Shred cheese using largest holes on box grater. If purchasing shredded cheese, look for "chef-style" cheese which is grated into larger than usual pieces.

1 Place mozzarella cheese in colander with large holes; shake to separate large shreds of cheese from smaller shreds; save smaller shreds for another use. Transfer large shreds of cheese to medium bowl; add Parmesan and toss to blend.

2 Remove white ends from green onions. Slit open onions lengthwise with paring knife and then thinly slice crosswise. Add to bowl with cheese. Add chili powder and pepper; toss gently.

3 Spray medium nonstick skillet with cooking spray; heat over medium-high heat. Sprinkle about 1 tablespoon cheese mixture in single layer in skillet making lacy 2-inch circle. Cook 1 to 1½ minutes until cheese melts and turns golden brown. Immediately remove from pan with thin metal spatula; cool completely on parchment-lined baking sheet. Repeat with remaining cheese mixture.

NOTE

Cheese crisps are extremely hot and pliable when they are first removed from the skillet but become crispy and chewy as they cool. You can easily mold them by draping them over a rolling pin.

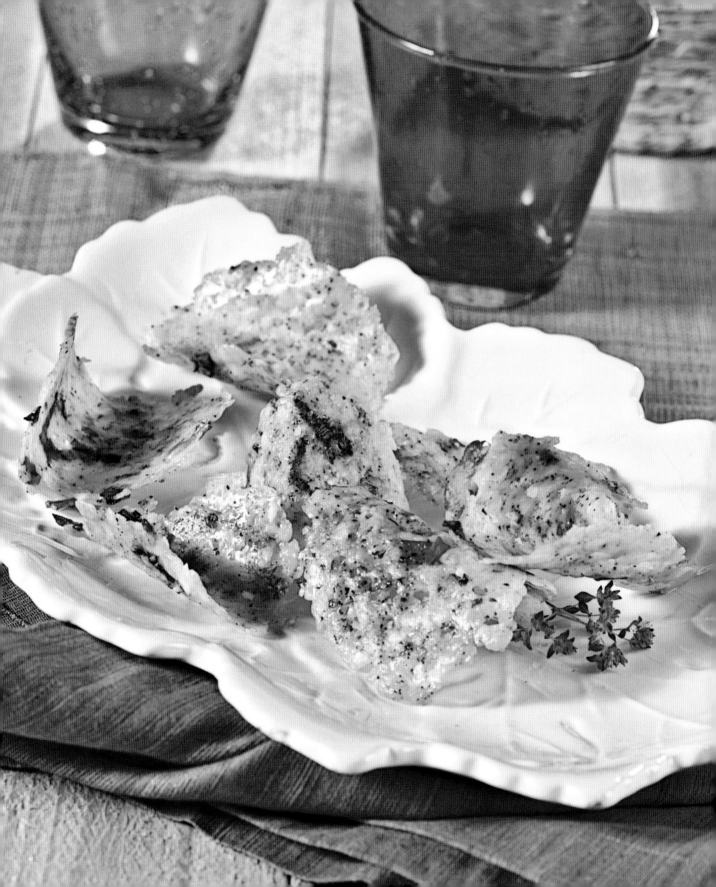

Beefy Stuffed Mushrooms

MAKES 18 MUSHROOMS

NUTRIENTS PER SERVING

CALORIES
40

TOTAL FAT
1g

SATURATED FAT
0g

CHOLESTEROL
13mg

SODIUM
20mg

CARBOHYDRATE
1g

DIETARY FIBER
0g

PROTEIN
6g

1 pound 90% lean ground beef

2 teaspoons prepared horseradish

1 teaspoon chopped fresh chives

1 clove garlic, minced

¼ teaspoon black pepper

18 large mushrooms

⅔ cup dry white wine

1 Preheat oven to 350°F. Combine beef, horseradish, chives, garlic and pepper in medium bowl; mix well.

2 Remove stems from mushrooms; fill caps with beef mixture.

3 Place stuffed mushrooms in shallow baking dish; pour wine over mushrooms. Bake 20 minutes or until meat is browned and cooked through.

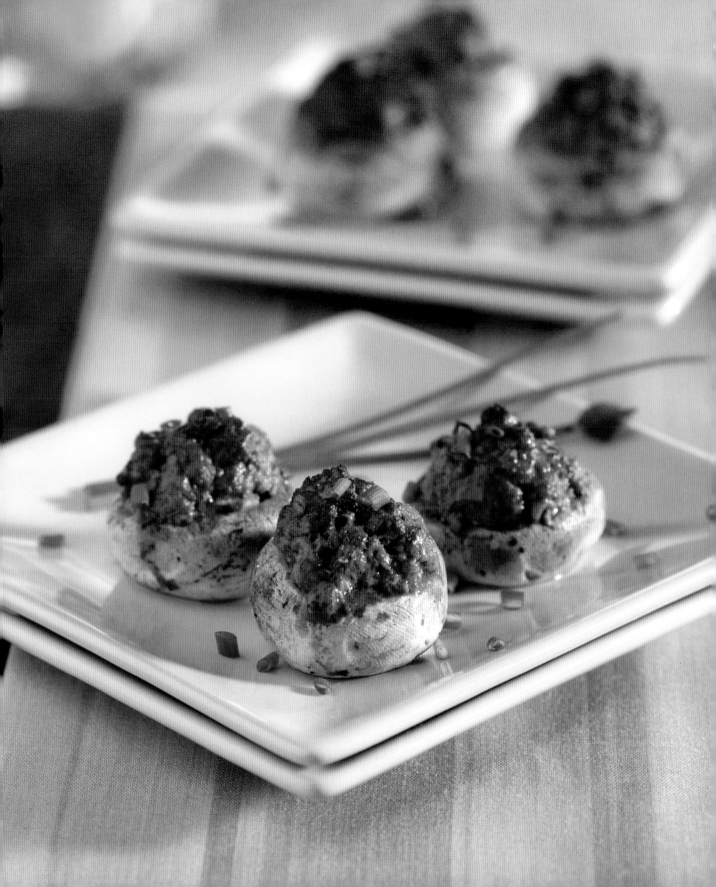

Paprika Almonds

MAKES ABOUT 8 SERVINGS (2 TABLESPOONS PER SERVING)

1 cup whole blanched almonds

¾ teaspoon olive oil

¼ teaspoon coarse salt

¼ teaspoon smoked paprika or paprika

1 Preheat oven to 375°F. Spread almonds in single layer in shallow baking pan. Bake 8 to 10 minutes or until almonds are lightly browned. Transfer to bowl; cool 5 to 10 minutes.

2 Toss almonds with oil until completely coated. Sprinkle with salt and paprika; toss again.

TIP

For the best flavor, serve these almonds the day they are made.

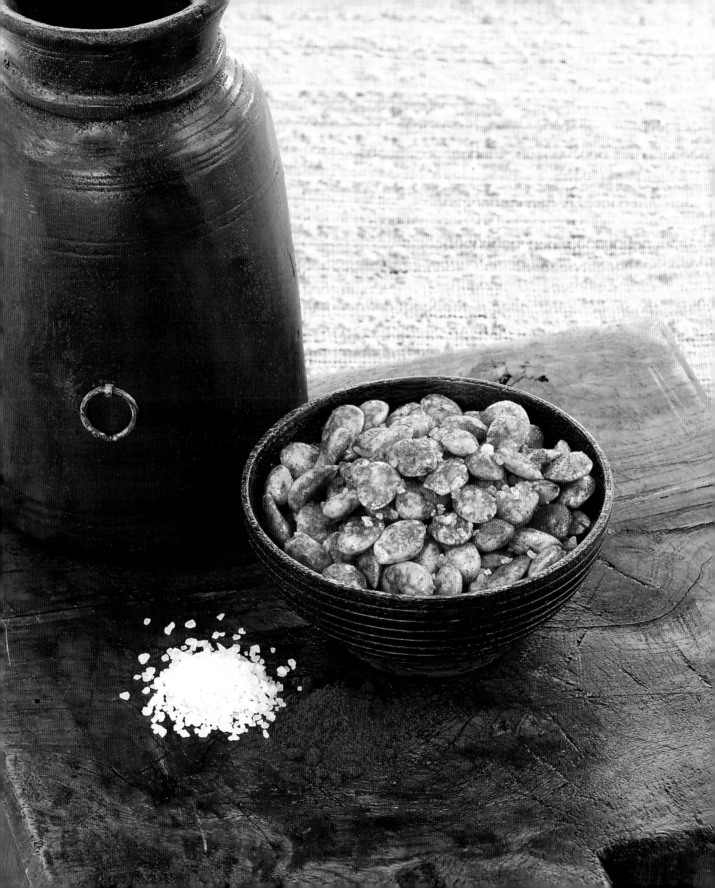

Spinach, Artichoke and Feta Dip

MAKES 6 SERVINGS (¼ CUP EACH)

NUTRIENTS PER SERVING

CALORIES
100

TOTAL FAT
7g

SATURATED FAT
4g

CHOLESTEROL
20mg

SODIUM
380mg

CARBOHYDRATE
6g

DIETARY FIBER
1g

PROTEIN
5g

½ cup thawed frozen chopped spinach

1 cup crumbled feta cheese

½ teaspoon black pepper

1 cup marinated artichokes, undrained

Cucumber slices and/or bell pepper strips

1 Place spinach in small microwavable bowl; microwave on HIGH 2 minutes.

2 Place cheese and pepper in food processor. Process 1 minute or until finely chopped. Add artichokes and spinach; process 30 seconds until well mixed but not puréed. Serve with vegetables.

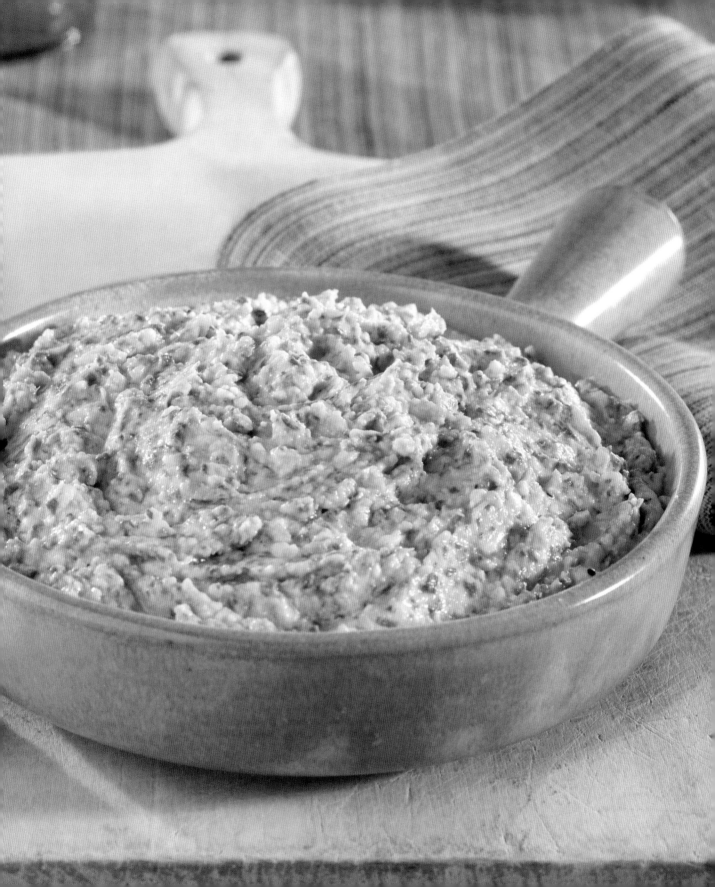

Lamb-Sicles

MAKES 4 SERVINGS

NUTRIENTS PER SERVING

CALORIES
370

TOTAL FAT
28g

SATURATED FAT
12g

CHOLESTEROL
90mg

SODIUM
670mg

CARBOHYDRATE
2g

DIETARY FIBER
0g

PROTEIN
29g

6 cloves garlic

1 teaspoon salt

2 tablespoons finely chopped fresh rosemary leaves

2 tablespoons olive oil

½ teaspoon ground black pepper

12 small lamb rib chops, bone-in and frenched*

The term frenched means that the fat and meat have been cut away from the end of the bone protruding from the chop. Ask the butcher to do this for you if frenched chops are not available already cut. You can also purchase a frenched rack of lamb and cut it into individual chops.

1 Chop garlic with salt until finely minced. Place in small bowl; add rosemary, oil and pepper. Mix well.

2 Rub mixture on both sides of lamb; wrap in single layer in foil and refrigerate 30 minutes to 3 hours.

3 Prepare grill for direct cooking or preheat broiler. Grill chops on well-oiled grid over medium-high heat 2 to 5 minutes per side or until medium-rare (145°F). Lamb should feel slightly firm when pressed. (To check doneness, cut small slit in meat near bone; lamb should be rosy pink.)

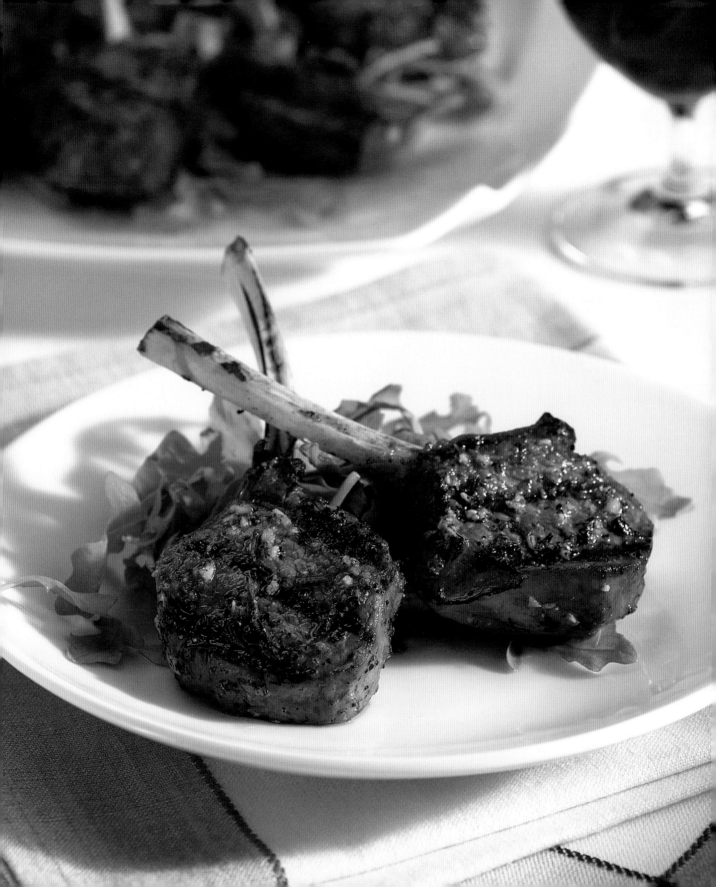

Kale Chips

MAKES 6 SERVINGS

1 large bunch kale (about 1 pound)
1 to 2 tablespoons olive oil

1 teaspoon garlic salt or other seasoned salt

1 Preheat oven to 350°F. Line baking sheets with parchment paper.

2 Wash kale and pat dry with paper towels. Remove center ribs and stems; discard. Cut leaves into 2- to 3-inch-wide pieces.

3 Combine leaves, oil and garlic salt in large bowl; toss to coat. Spread onto prepared baking sheets.

4 Bake 10 to 15 minutes or until edges are lightly browned and leaves are crisp.* Cool completely on baking sheets. Store in airtight container.

If the leaves are lightly browned but not crisp, turn oven off and let chips stand in oven until crisp, about 10 minutes. Do not keep the oven on as the chips will burn easily.

NUTRIENTS PER SERVING

CALORIES 43
TOTAL FAT 3g
SATURATED FAT 1g
CHOLESTEROL 0mg
SODIUM 180mg
CARBOHYDRATE 5g
DIETARY FIBER 1g
PROTEIN 2g

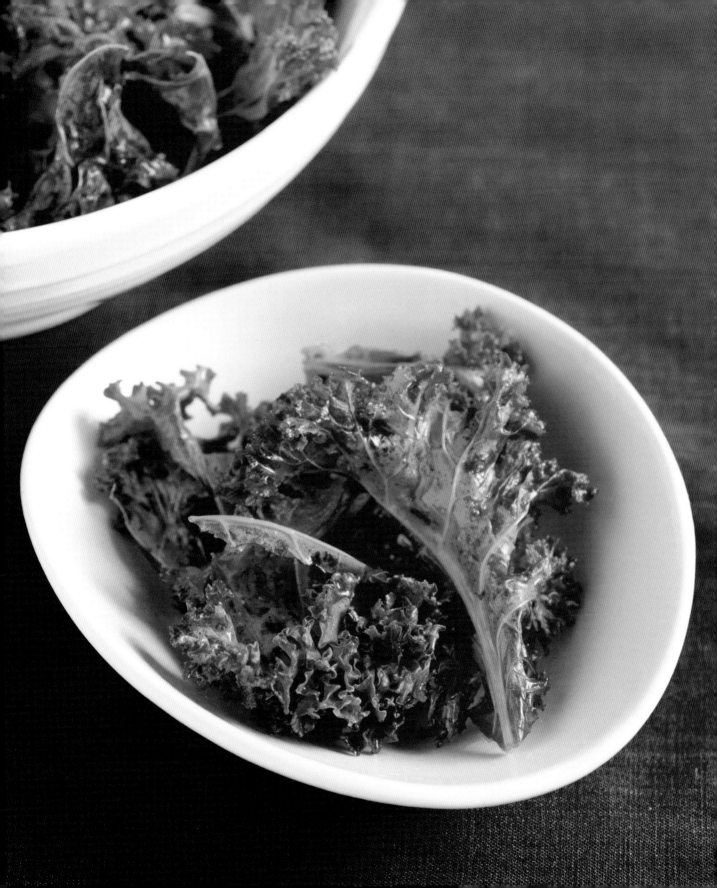

Rosemary-Scented Nut Mix

MAKES 6 CUPS (3 TABLESPOONS PER SERVING)

2 tablespoons unsalted butter

2 cups pecan halves

1 cup unsalted macadamia nuts

1 cup walnuts

1 teaspoon dried rosemary

½ teaspoon salt

¼ teaspoon red pepper flakes

1 Preheat oven to 300°F.

2 Melt butter in large saucepan over low heat. Stir in pecans, macadamia nuts and walnuts. Add rosemary, salt and red pepper flakes; cook and stir about 1 minute. Spread mixture onto ungreased baking sheet.

3 Bake 15 minutes, stirring occasionally. Cool completely on baking sheet on wire rack.

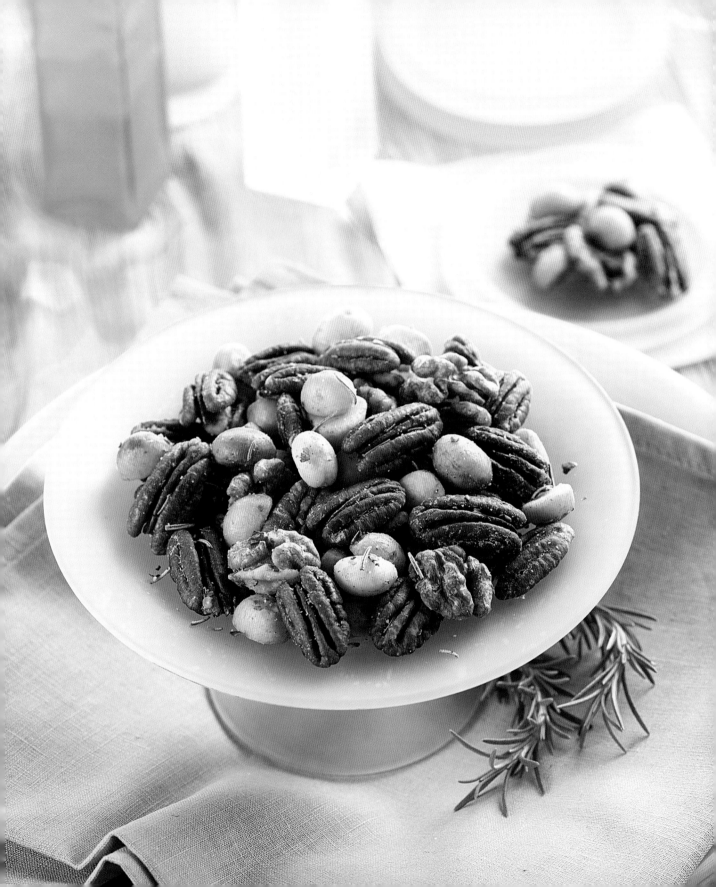

Zucchini Pizza Bites

MAKES 8 SERVINGS

1 medium zucchini

3 tablespoons pizza sauce

2 tablespoons tomato paste

¼ teaspoon dried oregano

¾ cup (3 ounces) shredded mozzarella cheese

¼ cup shredded Parmesan cheese

8 slices pitted black olives

8 slices pepperoni

1 Preheat broiler; set rack 4 inches from heat.

2 Trim off and discard ends of zucchini. Cut zucchini into 16 (¼-inch-thick) diagonal slices. Place on nonstick baking sheet.

3 Combine pizza sauce, tomato paste and oregano in small bowl; mix well. Spread scant teaspoon sauce over each zucchini slice. Combine cheeses in small bowl. Top each zucchini slice with 1 tablespoon cheese mixture, pressing down into sauce. Place 1 olive slice on each of 8 pizza bites. Place 1 folded pepperoni slice on each remaining pizza bite.

4 Broil 3 minutes or until cheese is melted. Serve immediately.

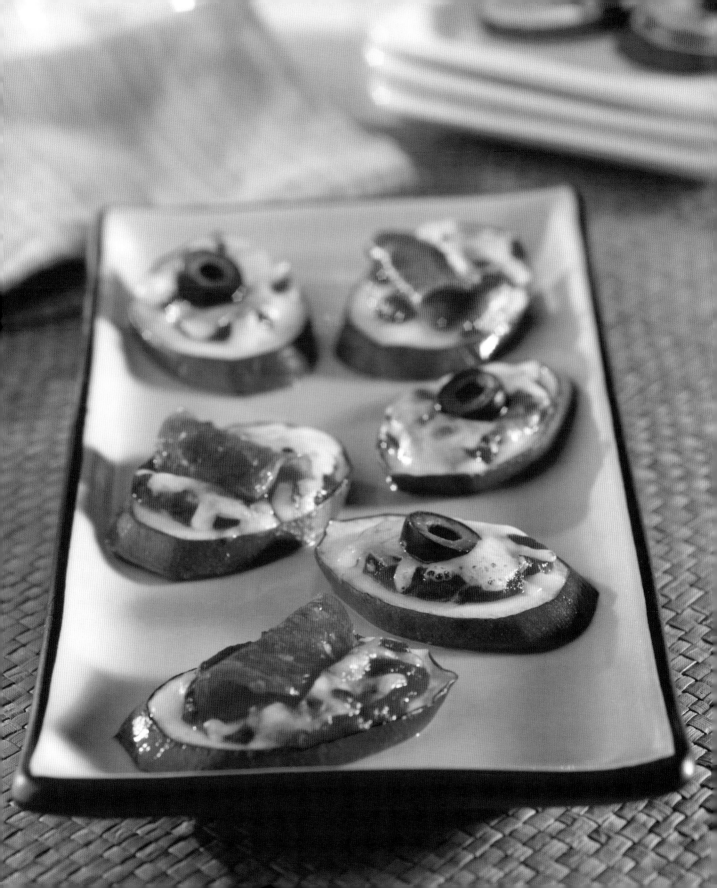

Mini Marinated Beef Skewers

MAKES 18 APPETIZERS

1 boneless beef top sirloin (about 1 pound)

2 tablespoons dry sherry

2 tablespoons soy sauce

1 tablespoon dark sesame oil

2 cloves garlic, minced

18 cherry tomatoes

Lettuce leaves (optional)

1 Cut beef crosswise into ⅛-inch slices. Place in large resealable food storage bag. Combine sherry, soy sauce, sesame oil and garlic in small bowl; pour over beef. Seal bag; turn to coat. Marinate in refrigerator at least 30 minutes or up to 2 hours. Soak 18 (6-inch) wooden skewers in water 20 minutes.

2 Preheat broiler. Drain beef; discard marinade. Weave beef accordion-style onto skewers. Place on rack of broiler pan.

3 Broil 4 to 5 inches from heat 2 minutes. Turn skewers over; broil 2 minutes or until beef is barely pink in center. Place 1 cherry tomato on each skewer. Serve warm or at room temperature.

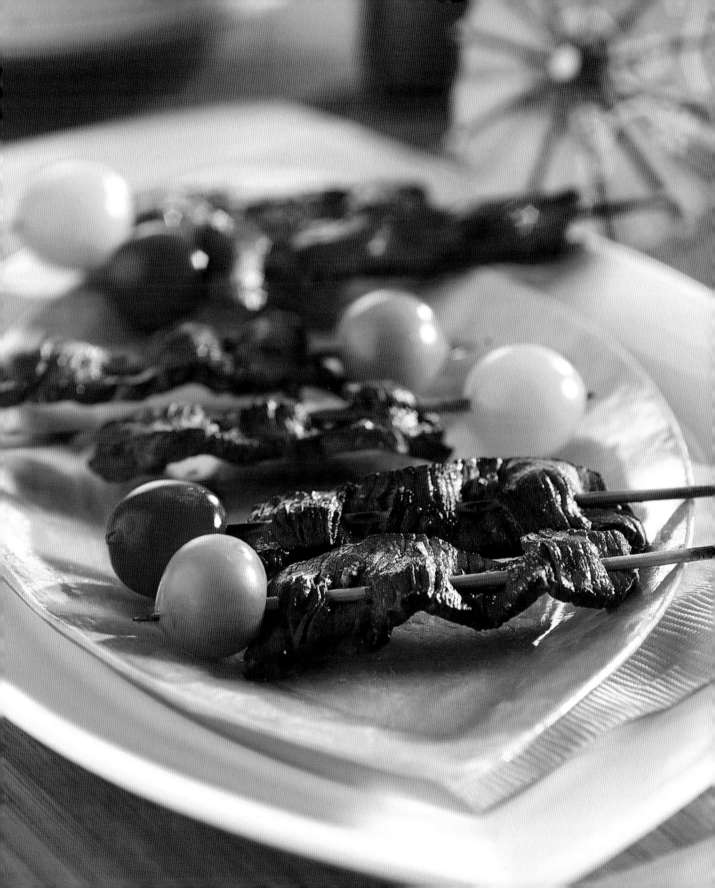

Spicy Deviled Eggs

MAKES 12 DEVILED EGGS (6 SERVINGS)

6 eggs

3 tablespoons whipping cream

1 green onion, finely chopped

1 tablespoon white wine vinegar

2 teaspoons Dijon mustard

½ teaspoon curry powder

½ teaspoon hot pepper sauce

Salt and black pepper

3 tablespoons crumbled crisp-cooked bacon

1 tablespoon chopped fresh chives

1 Bring medium saucepan of water to a boil over medium-high heat. Carefully add eggs; reduce heat to maintain a gentle boil. Cook 12 minutes. Drain and rinse under cold water. Peel eggs; cool completely.

2 Slice eggs in half lengthwise. Place yolks in small bowl; mash with fork. Stir in cream, green onion, vinegar, mustard, curry powder and hot pepper sauce until blended. Season to taste with salt and black pepper.

3 Spoon or pipe egg yolk mixture into centers of egg whites. Arrange eggs on serving plate. Sprinkle bacon over eggs. Garnish with chives.

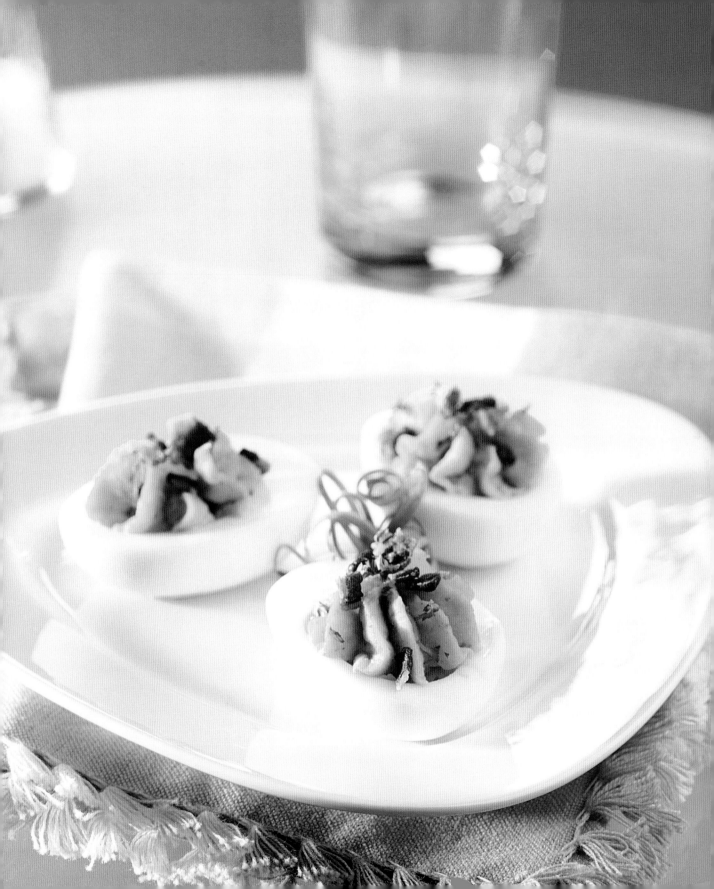

Parmesan-Pepper Crisps

MAKES ABOUT 26 CRISPS

NUTRIENTS PER SERVING

CALORIES
28

TOTAL FAT
2g

SATURATED FAT
1g

CHOLESTEROL
5mg

SODIUM
115mg

CARBOHYDRATE
1g

DIETARY FIBER
1g

PROTEIN
3g

2 cups loosely packed, coarsely grated Parmesan cheese

2 teaspoons black pepper

1 Preheat oven to 400°F. Line wire racks with paper towels.

2 Place heaping teaspoonfuls of cheese 2 inches apart on ungreased nonstick baking sheet. Flatten cheese mounds slightly with back of spoon. Sprinkle each mound with pinch of pepper.

3 Bake 15 to 20 minutes or until crisps are very lightly browned. (Watch closely; crisps burn easily.) Cool 2 minutes on baking sheet. Carefully remove with spatula to prepared racks. Store in airtight container in refrigerator up to 3 days.

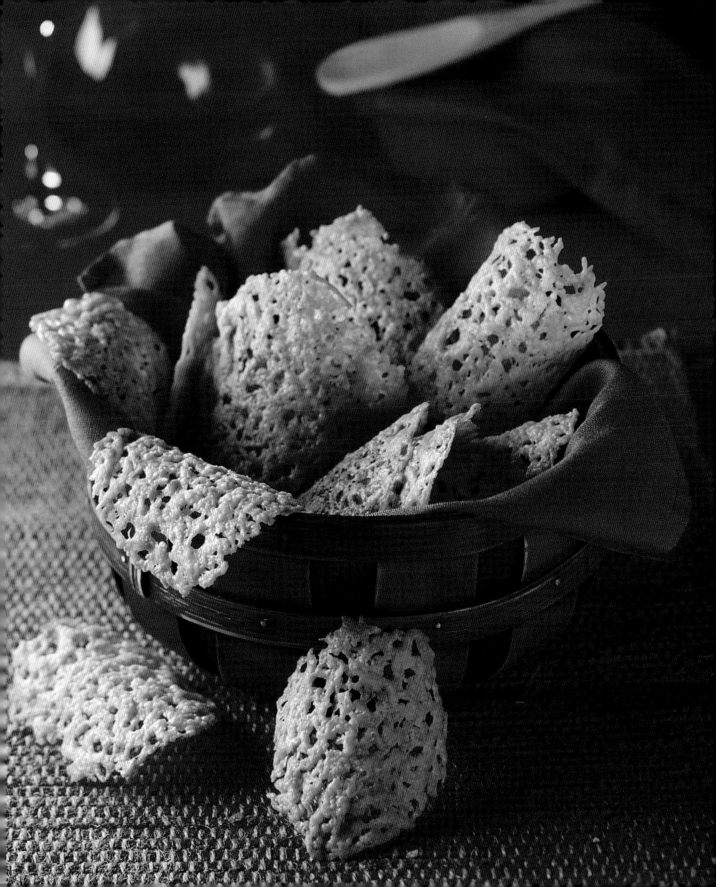

LUNCH

NUTRIENTS PER SERVING

CALORIES
145

TOTAL FAT
7g

SATURATED FAT
1g

CHOLESTEROL
38mg

SODIUM
285mg

CARBOHYDRATE
4g

DIETARY FIBER
0g

PROTEIN
16g

Spiced Chicken Skewers with Yogurt-Tahini Sauce

MAKES 8 SERVINGS

1 cup plain nonfat or regular Greek yogurt

¼ cup chopped fresh parsley, plus additional for garnish

¼ cup tahini

2 tablespoons lemon juice

1 clove garlic

¾ teaspoon salt, divided

1 tablespoon vegetable oil

2 teaspoons garam masala

1 pound boneless skinless chicken breasts, cut into 1-inch pieces

1 Spray grid with nonstick cooking spray. Prepare grill for direct cooking or preheat broiler.

2 For yogurt-tahini sauce, combine yogurt, ¼ cup parsley, tahini, lemon juice, garlic and ¼ teaspoon salt in food processor or blender; process until combined. Set aside.

3 Combine oil, garam masala and remaining ½ teaspoon salt in medium bowl. Add chicken; toss to coat evenly. Thread chicken on 8 (6-inch) metal or wooden skewers.*

4 Grill chicken skewers over medium-high heat or broil 5 minutes per side or until chicken is no longer pink. Serve with yogurt-tahini sauce; garnish with additional parsley.

If using wooden skewers, soak in cold water 20 minutes to prevent burning.

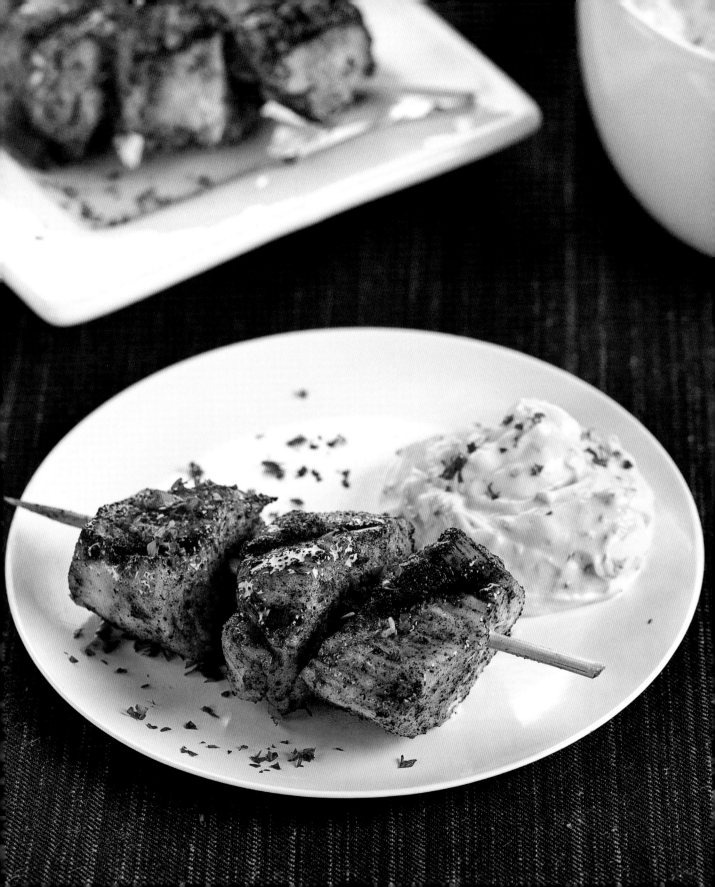

Veggie-Packed Pizza

MAKES 6 SERVINGS (1 WEDGE EACH)

2½ cups finely chopped fresh cauliflower (about ½ head)*

1½ cups (6 ounces) shredded part-skim mozzarella cheese, divided

1 egg

4 teaspoons chopped fresh oregano,** divided

½ cup sliced mushrooms

½ cup sliced assorted bell peppers (red, yellow, green and/or a combination)

½ cup sliced red onion

2 teaspoons olive oil

3 tablespoons pasta sauce or tomato sauce

Dash red pepper flakes

*To chop cauliflower easily, place in food processor and pulse until finely chopped.

**Or use 1¼ teaspoons dried oregano. Use 1 teaspoon in step 3 and ¼ teaspoon in step 6.

1 Preheat oven to 450°F. Spray pizza pan with nonstick cooking spray. Line large baking sheet with foil.

2 Place cauliflower in medium microwavable bowl; microwave on HIGH 4 minutes. Stir; microwave on HIGH 4 minutes or until tender. Let cool slightly.

3 Add 1 cup cheese, egg and 2 teaspoons oregano to cauliflower; mix well. Pat mixture into 9-inch circle in prepared pizza pan; spray with cooking spray.

4 Combine mushrooms, bell peppers and onion on prepared baking sheet. Drizzle with oil; toss to coat.

5 Roast vegetables 14 to 15 minutes or until tender. Bake cauliflower crust during last 10 to 12 minutes of cooking time or until golden brown around edges.

6 Spread pasta sauce over crust; top with roasted vegetables and remaining ½ cup cheese. Bake 6 to 7 minutes or just until cheese is melted. Sprinkle with remaining 2 teaspoons oregano and red pepper flakes. Cut into 6 wedges.

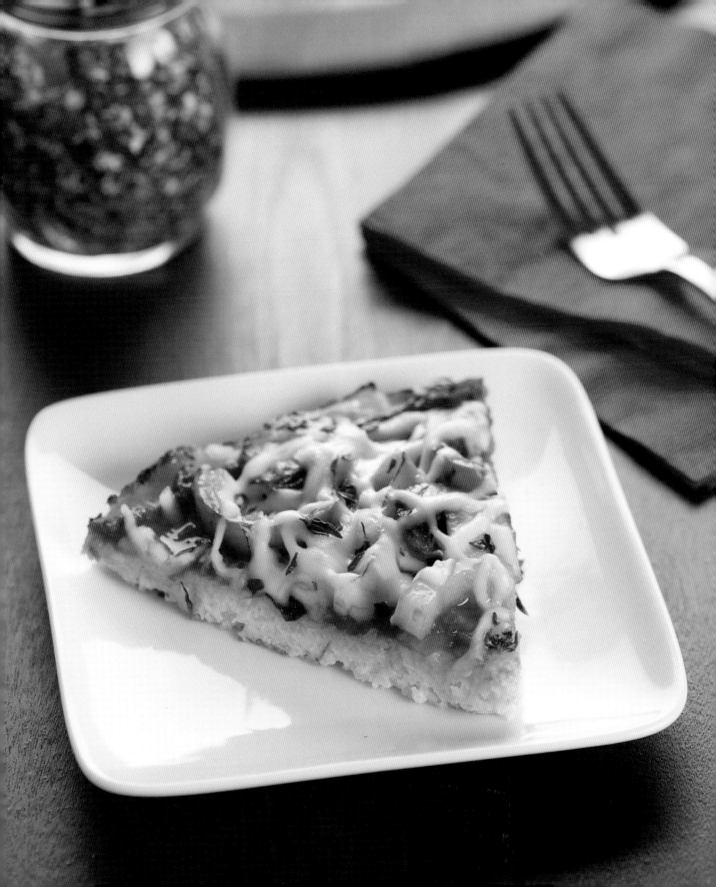

Egg White Salad Cucumber Boats

MAKES 2 SERVINGS

NUTRIENTS PER SERVING

CALORIES
175

TOTAL FAT
9g

SATURATED FAT
1g

CHOLESTEROL
6mg

SODIUM
756mg

CARBOHYDRATE
11g

DIETARY FIBER
1g

PROTEIN
12g

6 hard-cooked eggs, peeled

⅓ cup light or regular mayonnaise

Juice of 1 lemon

1 teaspoon chopped fresh dill

¼ teaspoon salt

¼ cup finely chopped green bell pepper

¼ cup finely chopped red bell pepper

2 tablespoons finely chopped red onion

1 English cucumber

1 Slice eggs in half lengthwise; discard yolks. Finely grate or chop egg whites.

2 Whisk mayonnaise, lemon juice, 1 teaspoon dill and salt in medium bowl. Gently stir in egg whites, bell peppers and onion.

3 Cut cucumber in half crosswise; cut each piece in half lengthwise to make 4 equal pieces. Scoop out cucumber pieces with rounded ½ teaspoon, leaving thick shell. Fill each shell evenly with egg salad.

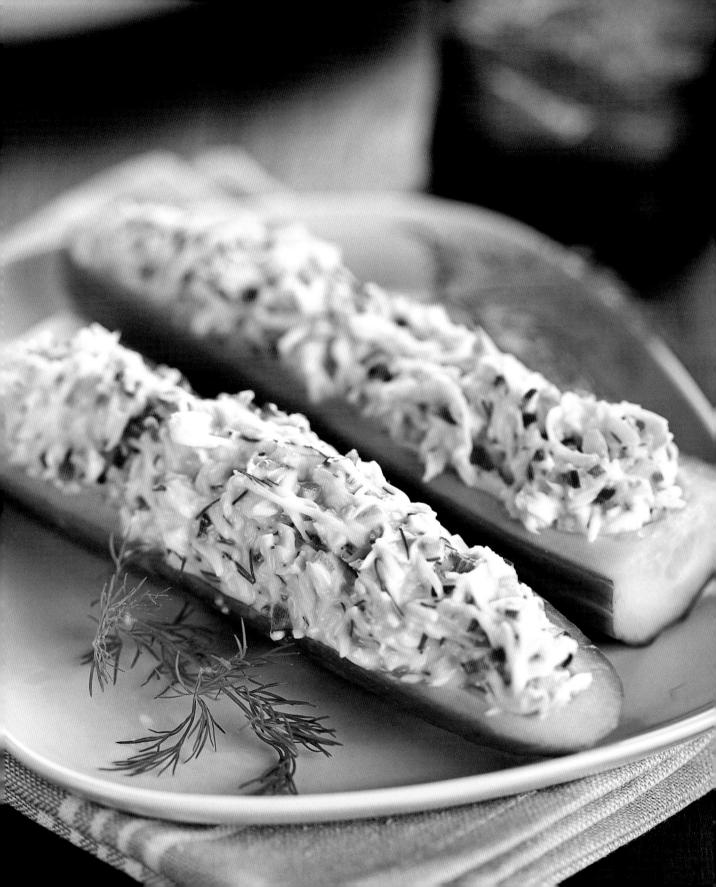

Spicy Chicken Bundles

MAKES 12 BUNDLES

NUTRIENTS PER SERVING

CALORIES
90

TOTAL FAT
6g

SATURATED FAT
2g

CHOLESTEROL
35mg

SODIUM
25mg

CARBOHYDRATE
3g

DIETARY FIBER
1g

PROTEIN
8g

1 pound ground chicken or turkey

2 teaspoons minced fresh ginger

2 cloves garlic, minced

¼ teaspoon red pepper flakes

1 tablespoon peanut or vegetable oil

3 tablespoons soy sauce

⅓ cup finely chopped water chestnuts

⅓ cup thinly sliced green onions

¼ cup chopped peanuts

12 large lettuce leaves, such as romaine

Chinese hot mustard (optional)

1 Combine chicken, ginger, garlic and red pepper flakes in medium bowl.

2 Heat oil in wok or large skillet over medium-high heat. Add chicken mixture; cook and stir 2 to 3 minutes until chicken is cooked through.

3 Add soy sauce; stir-fry 30 seconds. Add water chestnuts, green onions and peanuts; heat through.*

4 Divide filling evenly among lettuce leaves; roll up. Secure with toothpicks. Serve warm or at room temperature. Do not let filling stand at room temperature more than 2 hours. Serve with hot mustard, if desired.

Filling may be made ahead to this point; cover and refrigerate. Just before serving, reheat filling until warm. Proceed as directed in step 4.

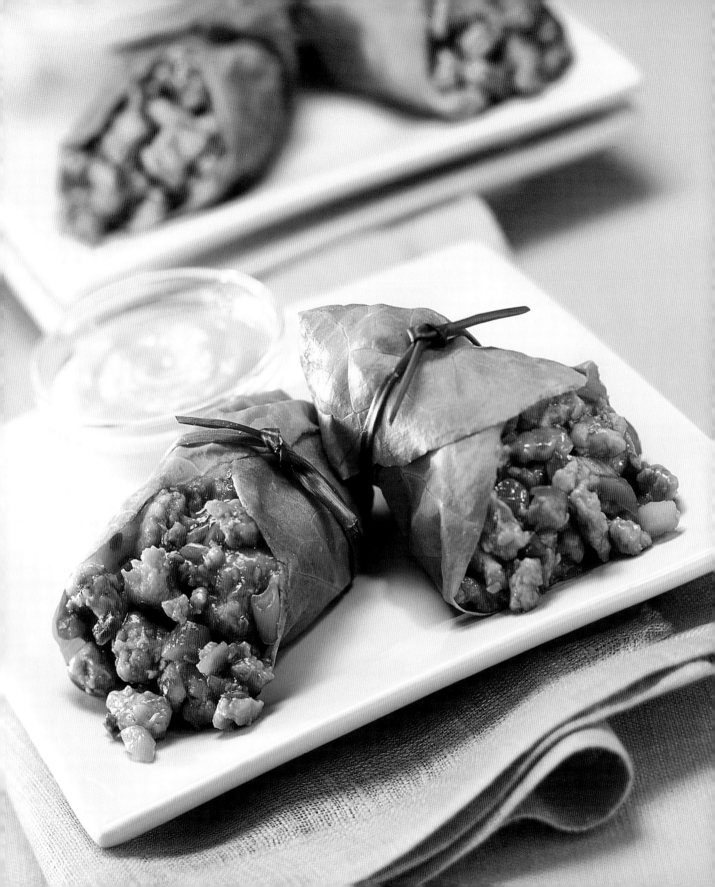

Chorizo and Caramelized Onion Tortilla

MAKES 36 SQUARES

NUTRIENTS PER SERVING	
CALORIES	100
TOTAL FAT	8g
SATURATED FAT	3g
CHOLESTEROL	75mg
SODIUM	180mg
CARBOHYDRATE	2g
DIETARY FIBER	0g
PROTEIN	5g

¼ cup olive oil

3 medium yellow onions, quartered and sliced

8 ounces Spanish chorizo (about 2 links) or andouille sausage, diced

6 eggs

Salt and black pepper

½ cup chopped fresh parsley

1 Heat oil in medium skillet over medium heat. Add onions; cover and cook 10 minutes or until translucent. Reduce heat to low; cook, uncovered, 40 minutes or until onions are golden brown and very tender, stirring occasionally. Remove onions from skillet and set aside to cool.

2 Add chorizo to same skillet. Cook over medium heat 5 minutes or just until chorizo begins to brown, stirring occasionally. Remove chorizo from skillet; set aside to cool.

3 Preheat oven to 350°F. Spray 9-inch square baking pan with olive oil cooking spray.

4 Whisk eggs in medium bowl; season with salt and pepper. Add onions, chorizo and parsley; stir gently until well blended. Pour into prepared pan.

5 Bake 12 to 15 minutes or until center is almost set. Turn oven to broil. Broil 1 to 2 minutes or until top just starts to brown. Transfer pan to wire rack; cool completely. Cut into 36 triangles or squares; serve cold or at room temperature.

TIP

The tortilla can be made up to 1 day ahead and refrigerated until serving. To serve at room temperature, remove from refrigerator 30 minutes before serving.

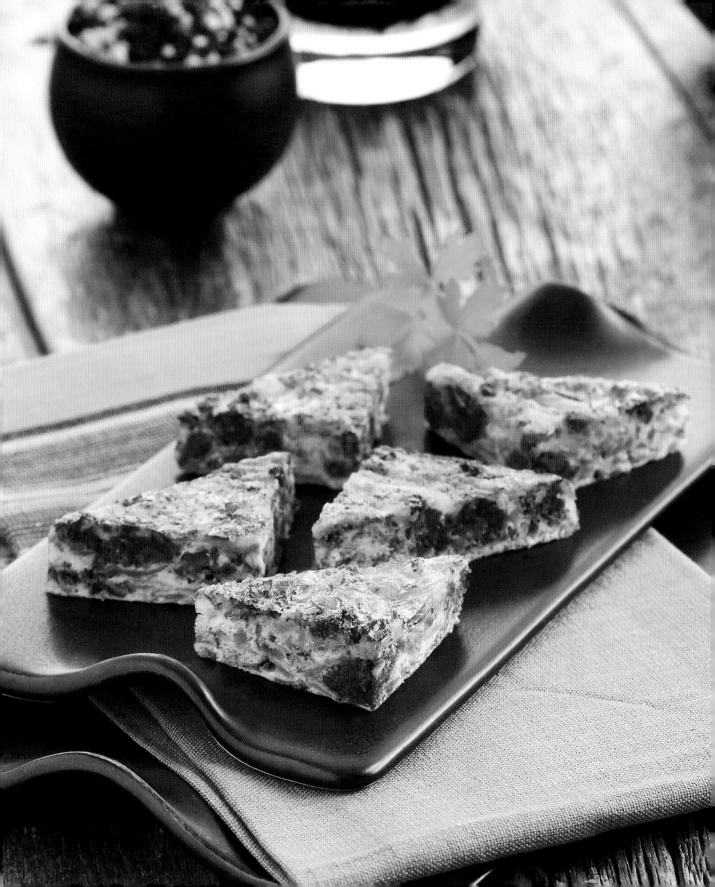

Chicken Avocado Boats

MAKES 6 SERVINGS

3 large ripe avocados, cut in half and pitted

6 tablespoons lemon juice

¾ cup mayonnaise

1½ tablespoons grated onion

¼ teaspoon celery salt

¼ teaspoon garlic powder

Salt and black pepper

2 cups diced cooked chicken

½ cup (2 ounces) shredded sharp Cheddar cheese

1 Preheat oven to 350°F. Sprinkle each avocado half with 1 tablespoon lemon juice; set aside.

2 Combine mayonnaise, onion, celery salt and garlic powder in medium bowl. Stir in chicken; mix well. Season with salt and pepper.

3 Drain any excess lemon juice from avocado halves. Fill avocado halves with chicken mixture; sprinkle with cheese.

4 Arrange filled avocado halves in single layer in baking dish. Pour water into same dish to depth of ½ inch. Bake 15 minutes or until cheese melts.

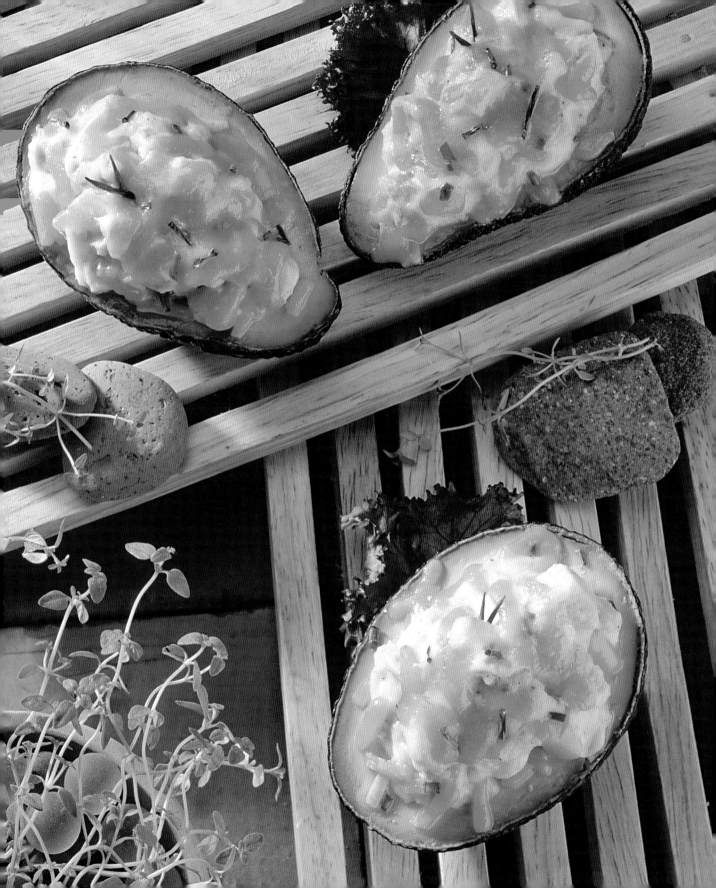

Poblano Pepper Kabobs

MAKES 4 SERVINGS

NUTRIENTS PER SERVING

CALORIES
145

TOTAL FAT
9g

SATURATED FAT
6g

CHOLESTEROL
43mg

SODIUM
532mg

CARBOHYDRATE
3g

DIETARY FIBER
1g

PROTEIN
13g

1 large poblano pepper

4 ounces smoked turkey breast, cut into 8 cubes

4 ounces pepper jack cheese, cut into 8 cubes

¼ cup salsa (optional)

1 Preheat oven to 400°F. Fill medium saucepan half full with water; bring to a boil over medium-high heat. Add poblano pepper; cook 1 minute. Cut pepper into 12 pieces when cool enough to handle.

2 Alternately thread pepper, turkey and cheese onto 4 short wooden skewers.

3 Place kabobs on baking sheet. Bake 3 minutes or until cheese starts to melt. Serve with salsa, if desired.

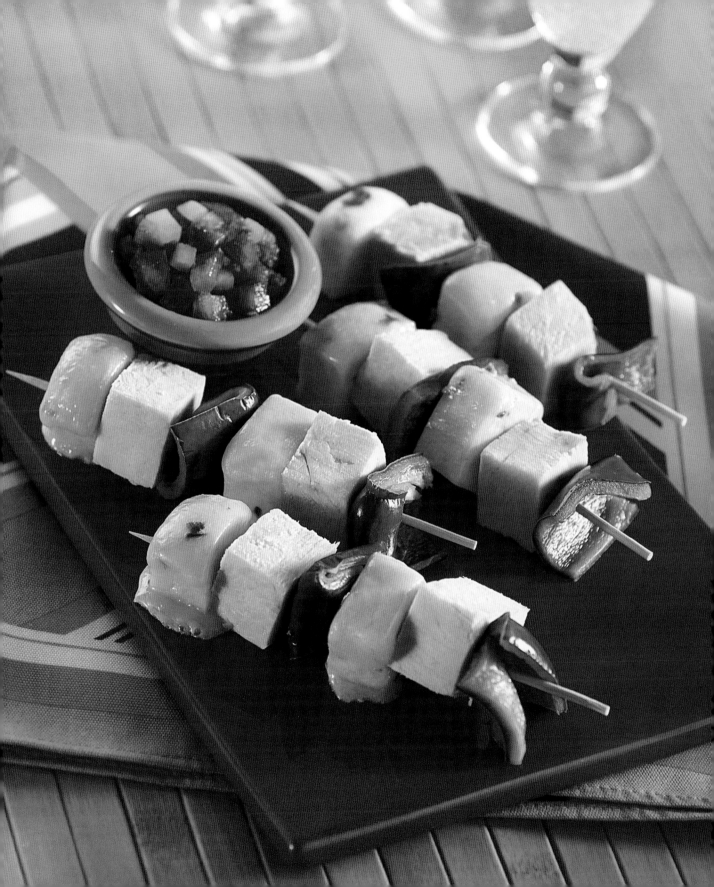

Hot or Cold Tuna Snacks

MAKES 6 SERVINGS (3 PIECES EACH)

**NUTRIENTS
PER SERVING**

CALORIES
83

TOTAL FAT
5g

SATURATED FAT
2g

CHOLESTEROL
21mg

SODIUM
196mg

CARBOHYDRATE
2g

DIETARY FIBER
1g

PROTEIN
9g

1 can (6 ounces) water-packed chunk light tuna, drained

4 ounces reduced-fat or regular cream cheese, softened

1 tablespoon chopped fresh parsley

1 tablespoon minced onion

½ teaspoon dried oregano

½ teaspoon black pepper

18 (½-inch-thick) slices seedless cucumber

18 capers (optional)

1 Combine tuna, cream cheese, parsley, onion, oregano and pepper in medium bowl; mix well.

2 Mound about 1 tablespoon tuna mixture on top of each cucumber slice. To serve cold, garnish with capers and serve immediately.

3 To serve hot, preheat oven to 450°F. Spray baking sheet with nonstick cooking spray. Place snacks on prepared baking sheet; bake about 10 minutes or until tops are puffed and brown. Garnish with capers.

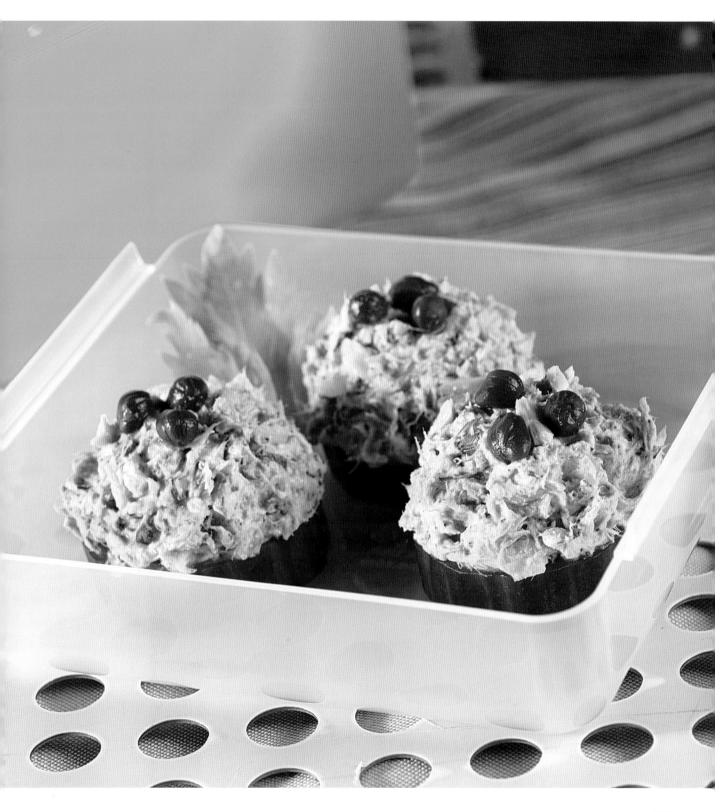

Ham and Cheese Rolls

MAKES 8 SERVINGS (8 PIECES PER SERVING)

NUTRIENTS PER SERVING

CALORIES
145

TOTAL FAT
13g

SATURATED FAT
12g

CHOLESTEROL
40mg

SODIUM
263mg

CARBOHYDRATE
3g

DIETARY FIBER
1g

PROTEIN
5g

4 thin slices deli ham (4×4 inches)

1 package (8 ounces) cream cheese, softened

1 piece (4 inches long) seedless cucumber, quartered lengthwise (about ½ cucumber)

4 thin slices American or Cheddar cheese (4×4 inches), at room temperature

1 red bell pepper, cut into thin 4-inch-long strips

1 For ham sushi, pat 1 ham slice with paper towel to remove excess moisture and place on cutting board. Spread 2 tablespoons cream cheese to edges of ham slice. Pat 1 cucumber piece with paper towel to remove excess moisture; place at edge of ham slice. Roll up tightly, pressing gently to seal. Wrap in plastic wrap; refrigerate. Repeat with remaining ham slices, cream cheese and cucumber pieces.

2 For cheese sushi, spread 2 tablespoons cream cheese to edges of 1 cheese slice. Place 2 red pepper strips at edge of cheese slice. Roll up tightly, pressing gently to seal. Wrap in plastic wrap; refrigerate. Repeat with remaining cheese slices, cream cheese and red pepper strips.

3 To serve, remove plastic wrap from ham and cheese rolls. Cut each roll into 8 (½-inch-wide) pieces.

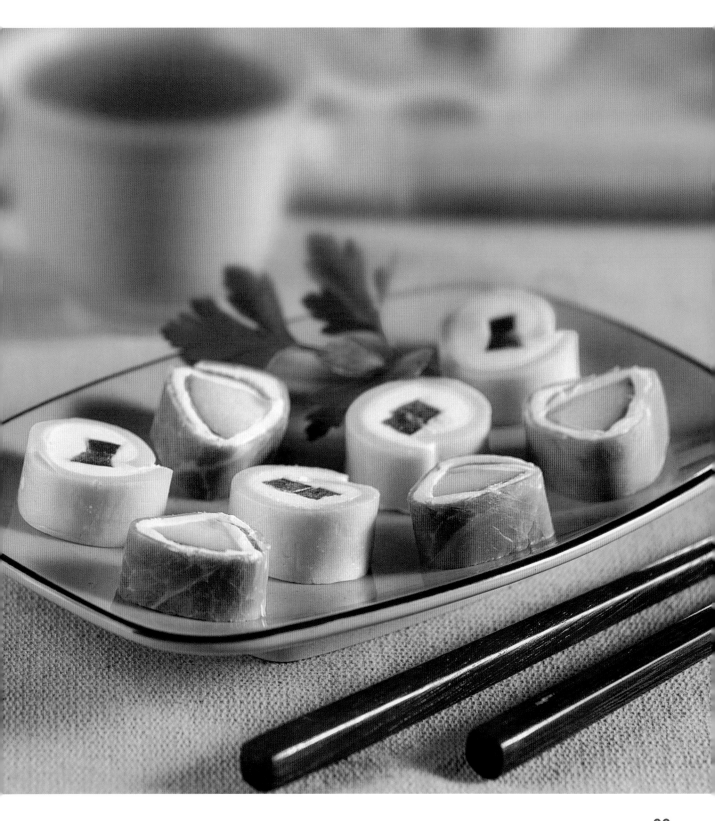

Roast Beef Roll-Ups

MAKES 2 SERVINGS

2 tablespoons horseradish mayonnaise

2 thin slices roast beef (1 ounce)

¼ cup (1 ounce) crumbled blue cheese

1 ounce sliced red onion

1 Spread mayonnaise on roast beef slices. Sprinkle with blue cheese; layer with onion slices.

2 Roll up roast beef slices from short ends.

NUTRIENTS PER SERVING

CALORIES
80

TOTAL FAT
5g

SATURATED FAT
1g

CHOLESTEROL
14mg

SODIUM
365mg

CARBOHYDRATE
2g

DIETARY FIBER
1g

PROTEIN
6g

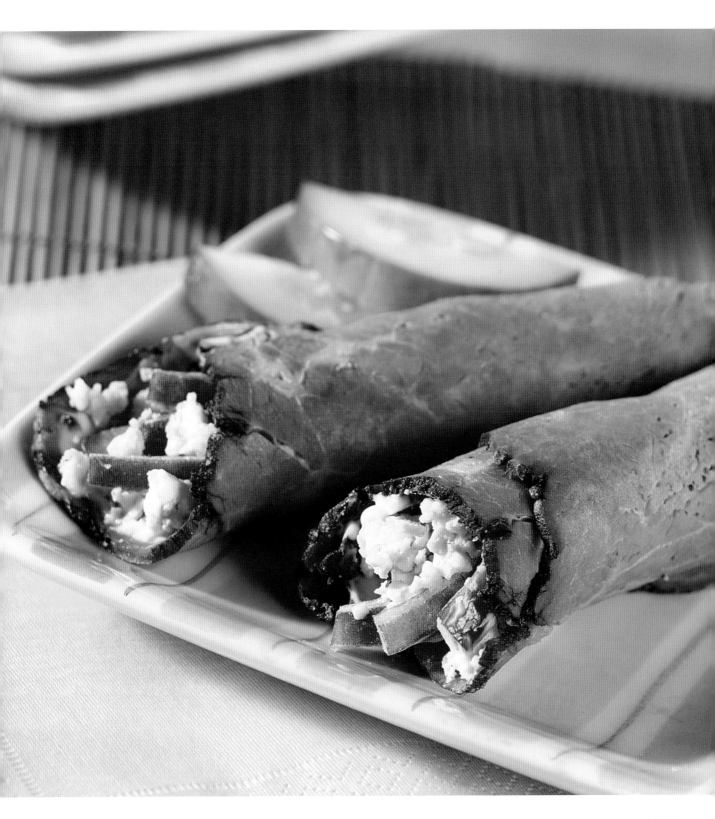

SALADS and SOUPS

Grilled Tri-Colored Pepper Salad

MAKES 4 TO 6 SERVINGS

1 *each* large red, yellow and green bell pepper, cut into halves or quarters

⅓ cup extra virgin olive oil

3 tablespoons balsamic vinegar

2 cloves garlic, minced

¼ teaspoon salt

¼ teaspoon black pepper

⅓ cup crumbled goat cheese (about 1½ ounces)

¼ cup thinly sliced fresh basil leaves

1 Prepare grill for direct cooking over high heat.

2 Place bell peppers, skin side down, on grid. Grill, covered, 10 to 12 minutes or until skin is charred. Transfer to paper bag. Close bag; let stand 10 to 15 minutes. Remove and discard skin. Place bell peppers in shallow serving dish.

3 Whisk oil, vinegar, garlic, salt and black pepper in small bowl until well blended. Pour over bell peppers. Let stand 30 minutes at room temperature. (Or cover and refrigerate up to 24 hours. Bring bell peppers to room temperature before serving.)

4 Sprinkle with goat cheese and basil just before serving.

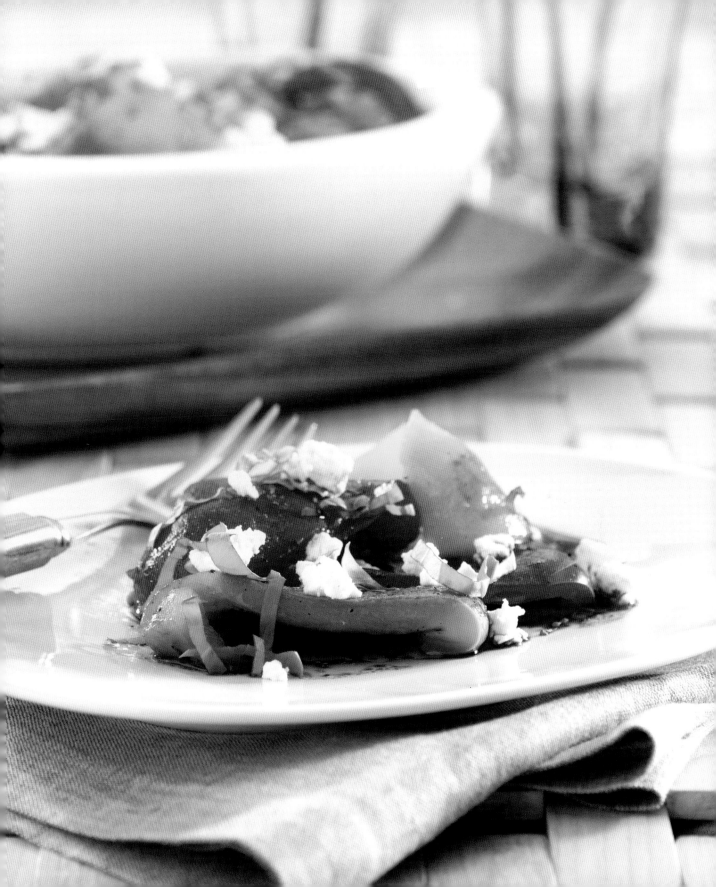

Tomato, Avocado and Cucumber Salad

MAKES 4 SERVINGS

**NUTRIENTS
PER SERVING**

CALORIES
138

TOTAL FAT
11g

SATURATED FAT
2g

CHOLESTEROL
3mg

SODIUM
311mg

CARBOHYDRATE
7g

DIETARY FIBER
2g

PROTEIN
4g

1½ tablespoons extra virgin olive oil

1 tablespoon balsamic vinegar

1 clove garlic, minced

¼ teaspoon salt

¼ teaspoon black pepper

2 cups diced seeded plum tomatoes

1 small ripe avocado, diced into ½-inch chunks

½ cup chopped cucumber

⅓ cup crumbled reduced-fat or regular feta cheese

4 large red leaf lettuce leaves

Chopped fresh basil

1 Whisk oil, vinegar, garlic, salt and pepper in medium bowl. Add tomatoes and avocado; toss to coat evenly. Gently stir in cucumber and feta cheese.

2 Arrange 1 lettuce leaf on each serving plate. Spoon salad evenly onto lettuce leaves. Sprinkle with basil.

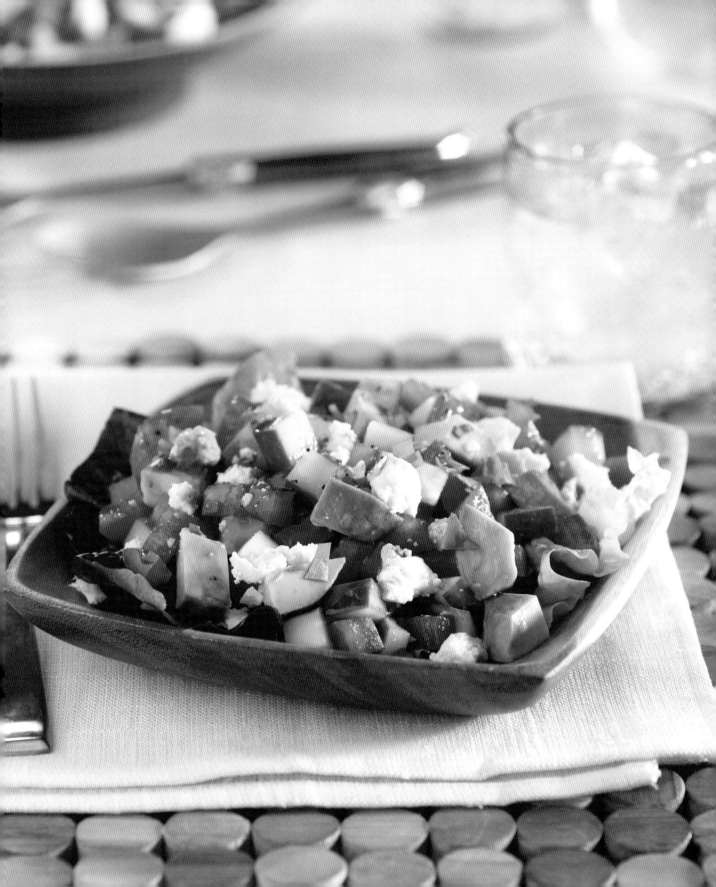

Cobb Salad

MAKES 4 SERVINGS

NUTRIENTS PER SERVING

CALORIES
350

TOTAL FAT
27g

SATURATED FAT
5g

CHOLESTEROL
35mg

SODIUM
1050mg

CARBOHYDRATE
11g

DIETARY FIBER
6g

PROTEIN
17g

1 package (10 ounces) mixed salad greens *or* 8 cups torn romaine lettuce

6 ounces deli chicken, turkey or smoked turkey, diced

1 large tomato, seeded and chopped

⅓ cup crisp-cooked and crumbled bacon

1 large ripe avocado, diced

¼ cup crumbled blue cheese

½ cup prepared blue cheese or Caesar salad dressing

1 Place salad greens in serving bowl. Arrange chicken, tomato, bacon and avocado in rows.

2 Sprinkle with blue cheese. Serve with dressing.

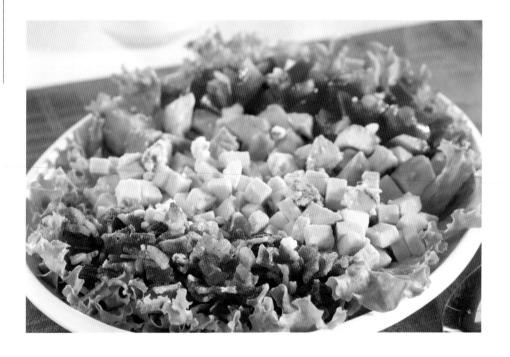

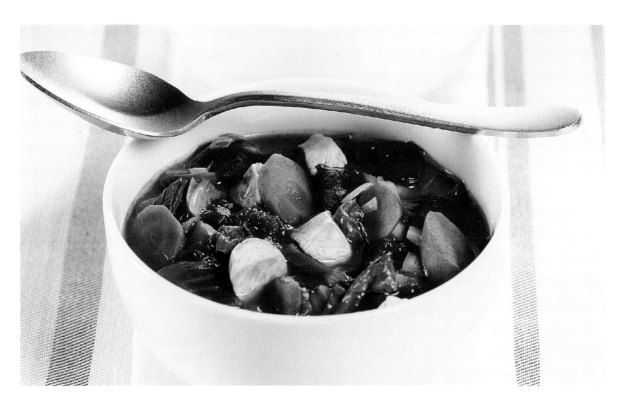

Chunky Chicken Stew

NUTRIENTS
PER SERVING

CALORIES
140

TOTAL FAT
4g

SATURATED FAT
0g

CHOLESTEROL
30mg

SODIUM
390mg

CARBOHYDRATE
13g

DIETARY FIBER
3g

PROTEIN
14g

MAKES 2 SERVINGS

1 teaspoon olive oil

1 small onion, chopped

½ cup thinly sliced carrots

1 cup reduced-sodium chicken broth

2 cups peeled diced plum tomatoes

1 cup diced cooked chicken breast (2 ounces)

3 cups sliced kale or baby spinach

1 Heat oil in large saucepan over medium-high heat. Add onion; cook and stir about 5 minutes or until golden brown. Stir in carrots and broth; bring to a boil. Reduce heat; simmer, uncovered, 5 minutes.

2 Stir in tomatoes; simmer 5 minutes or until carrots are tender. Add chicken; cook and stir until heated through. Add kale; stir until wilted.

Shrimp Gazpacho

MAKES 4 SERVINGS

NUTRIENTS PER SERVING

CALORIES
101

TOTAL FAT
3g

SATURATED FAT
0g

CHOLESTEROL
86mg

SODIUM
232mg

CARBOHYDRATE
8g

DIETARY FIBER
1g

PROTEIN
13g

- 1 teaspoon olive oil
- 8 ounces medium raw shrimp, peeled and deveined
- ¼ teaspoon salt (optional)
- ⅛ teaspoon black pepper
- 3 plum tomatoes, chopped (about 1½ cups)
- ¼ small red onion, chopped
- 1 clove garlic, chopped
- ¼ cucumber, peeled and chopped
- ¼ cup finely chopped jarred roasted red peppers, divided
- ¾ cup tomato juice
- 1 tablespoon red wine vinegar

1 Heat oil in medium nonstick skillet over high heat. Season shrimp with salt, if desired, and black pepper. Add to skillet; cook 3 minutes or until browned on both sides and opaque in center. Transfer to plate.

2 Combine tomatoes, onion, garlic, cucumber and half of roasted peppers in food processor; process until blended. Add tomato juice and vinegar; process until smooth.

3 Divide tomato mixture among bowls; top with shrimp and remaining roasted peppers.

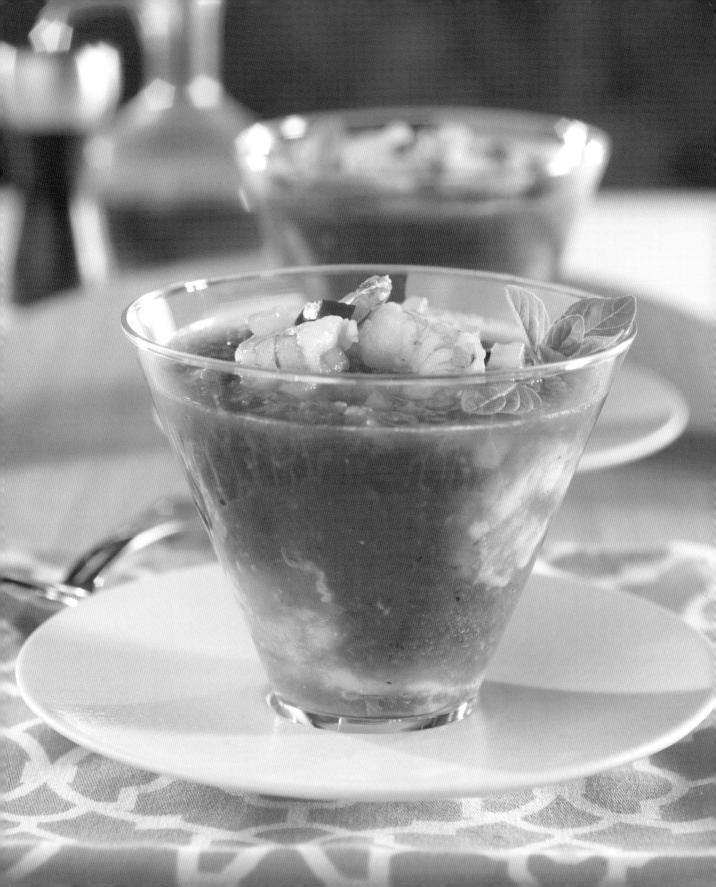

Greek-Style Kale and Sausage Stew

MAKES 6 SERVINGS

1 tablespoon olive oil

1 small onion, diced

1 pound uncooked Portuguese or hot Italian sausage

6 cups (4 ounces) coarsely chopped kale leaves (trimmed of thick stems)

1¼ cups hot chicken broth, divided

2 eggs, beaten

3 tablespoons fresh lemon juice

1 Heat oil in large saucepan. Add onion and cook over medium heat 5 minutes or until tender. Break sausage into bite-size pieces and add to pan. Brown sausage on all sides, about 5 minutes over medium heat, stirring frequently. Stir in kale and ½ cup broth. Cover, reduce heat and simmer 20 minutes or until kale is tender.

2 Whisk eggs and lemon juice in medium bowl. Whisking constantly, gradually add remaining ¾ cup hot broth to egg mixture. Pour egg mixture into kale and sausage mixture. Simmer over low heat 1 to 2 minutes or until egg mixture is slightly thickened. (Do not bring to a boil or eggs will scramble.)

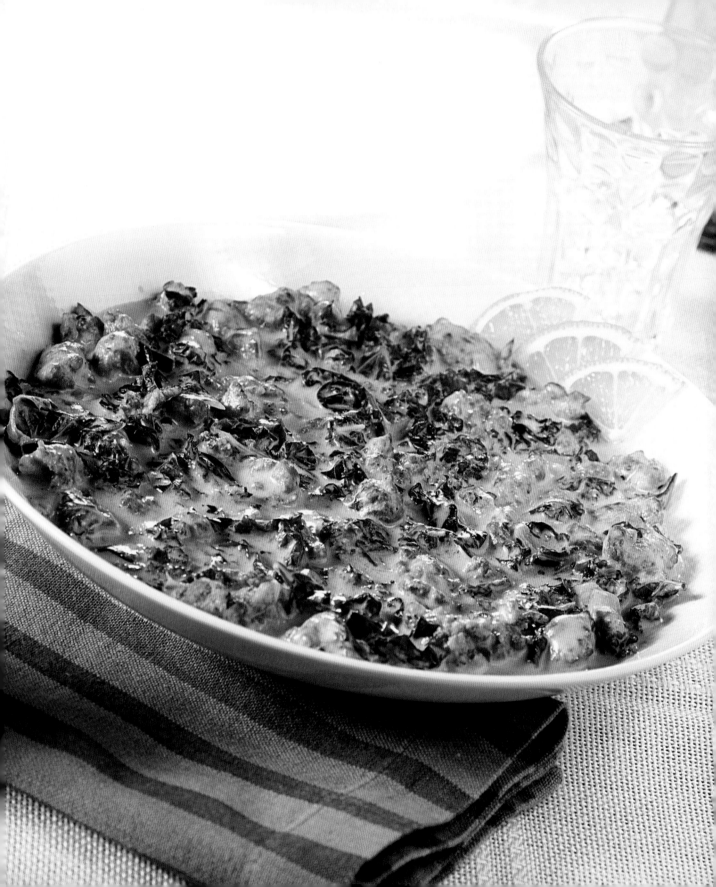

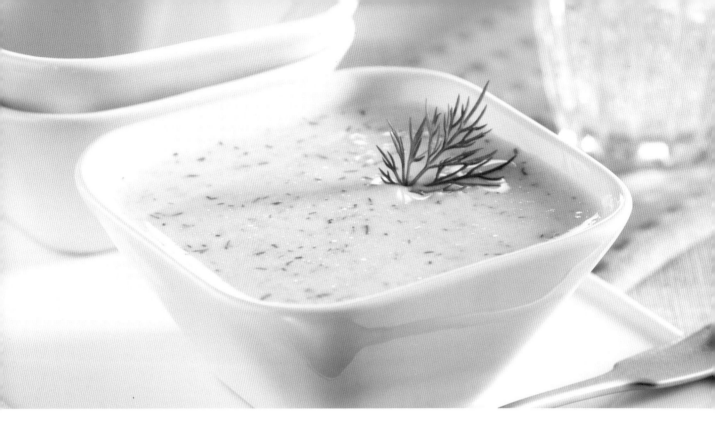

Chilled Cucumber Soup

MAKES 4 SERVINGS (¾ CUP PER SERVING)

NUTRIENTS
PER SERVING

CALORIES
67

TOTAL FAT
4g

SATURATED FAT
2g

CHOLESTEROL
13mg

SODIUM
236mg

CARBOHDRATE
6g

DIETARY FIBER
1g

PROTEIN
3g

1 large cucumber, peeled and coarsely chopped

¾ cup reduced-fat or regular sour cream

¼ cup packed fresh dill

½ teaspoon salt (optional)

⅛ teaspoon white pepper (optional)

1½ cups reduced-sodium chicken or vegetable broth

1 Place cucumber in food processor; process until finely chopped. Add sour cream, dill, salt and white pepper, if desired; process until fairly smooth.

2 Transfer mixture to large bowl; stir in broth. Cover and chill at least 2 hours or up to 24 hours.

Roasted Vegetable Salad

MAKES 4 SERVINGS

1 cup sliced mushrooms

¼ cup sliced carrots (optional)

1 cup chopped green or yellow bell pepper

1 cup cherry tomatoes, halved

½ cup chopped onion

2 tablespoons chopped pitted kalamata olives

2 teaspoons lemon juice, divided

1 teaspoon dried oregano

1 teaspoon olive oil

½ teaspoon black pepper

3 cups packed fresh spinach or baby spinach

1 Preheat oven to 375°F. Combine mushrooms, carrots, bell pepper, tomatoes, onion, olives, 1 teaspoon lemon juice, oregano, oil and black pepper in large bowl; toss to coat. Spread vegetables in single layer on baking sheet.

2 Roast 20 minutes, stirring once. Stir in remaining 1 teaspoon lemon juice. Serve warm over spinach.

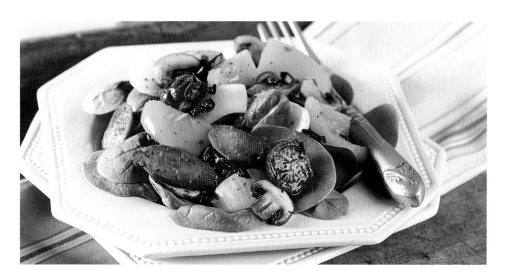

Southwestern Tuna Salad

MAKES 4 SERVINGS (1 CUP PER SERVING)

NUTRIENTS PER SERVING

CALORIES
180

TOTAL FAT
7g

SATURATED FAT
1g

CHOLESTEROL
32mg

SODIUM
185mg

CARBOHYDRATE
8g

DIETARY FIBER
3g

PROTEIN
21g

2 limes, juiced, divided

12 ounces raw tuna steaks (about 1 inch thick)

1 pint cherry or grape tomatoes, halved

¼ cup diced ripe avocado

1 jalapeño pepper, seeded and minced

1 green onion, chopped (green part only)

1 tablespoon chopped fresh cilantro

1½ teaspoons canola oil

¼ teaspoon salt

¼ teaspoon ground cumin

⅛ teaspoon black pepper

1 Place juice of one lime in glass baking dish or shallow bowl. Add tuna steaks. Marinate at room temperature 30 minutes, turning once.

2 Spray stovetop grill pan with nonstick cooking spray; heat over medium heat 30 seconds. Add tuna steaks; cook 5 to 6 minutes per side. Let cool to room temperature. Cut into bite-size chunks.

3 Combine tomatoes, avocado, jalapeño, green onion and cilantro in large bowl. Add tuna.

4 Whisk oil, remaining lime juice, salt, cumin and black pepper in small bowl. Pour over salad; toss to coat.

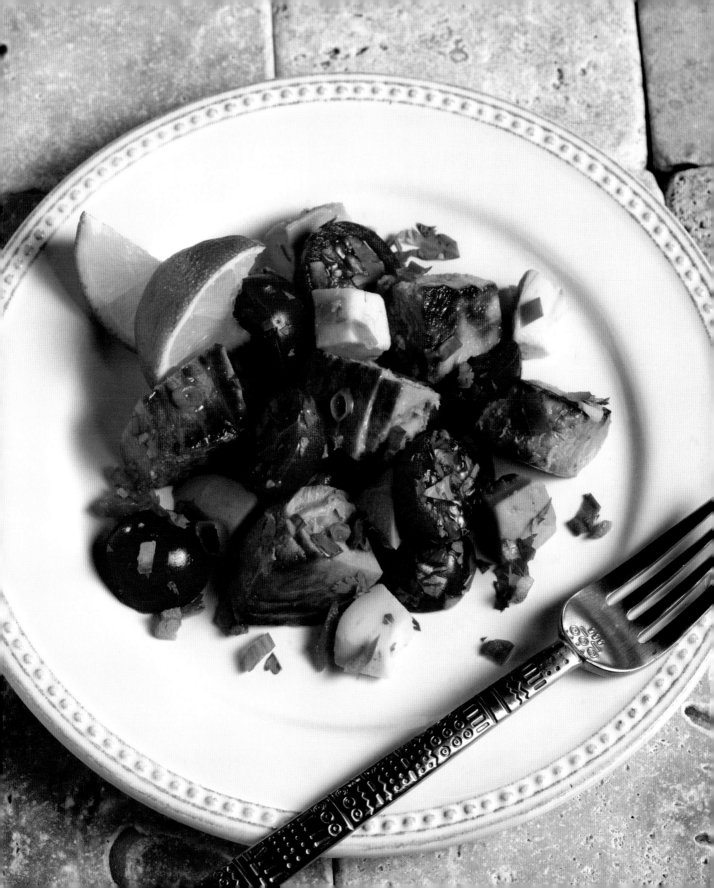

Mesclun Salad with Cranberry Vinaigrette

MAKES 4 SERVINGS

NUTRIENTS
PER SERVING

CALORIES
233

TOTAL FAT
19g

SATURATED FAT
5g

CHOLESTEROL
15mg

SODIUM
325mg

CARBOHYDRATE
10g

DIETARY FIBER
3g

PROTEIN
7g

DRESSING

- 3 tablespoons extra virgin olive oil
- 1½ tablespoons champagne vinegar or sherry vinegar
- 1½ teaspoons Dijon mustard
- ¼ teaspoon salt
- ⅛ teaspoon black pepper

SALAD

- 5 cups (5 ounces) mesclun or mixed torn salad greens
- 2 ounces goat cheese, crumbled
- ¼ cup dried cranberries
- ¼ cup walnuts or pecans, coarsely chopped and toasted*

To toast nuts, spread in single layer on baking sheet. Bake in preheated 350°F oven 8 to 10 minutes or until golden brown, stirring frequently.

1 For dressing, whisk oil, vinegar, mustard, salt and pepper in small bowl. Cover; refrigerate at least 30 minutes or up to 24 hours before serving.

2 For salad, combine salad greens, goat cheese, cranberries and walnuts in large bowl. Whisk dressing again and add to salad; toss until evenly coated.

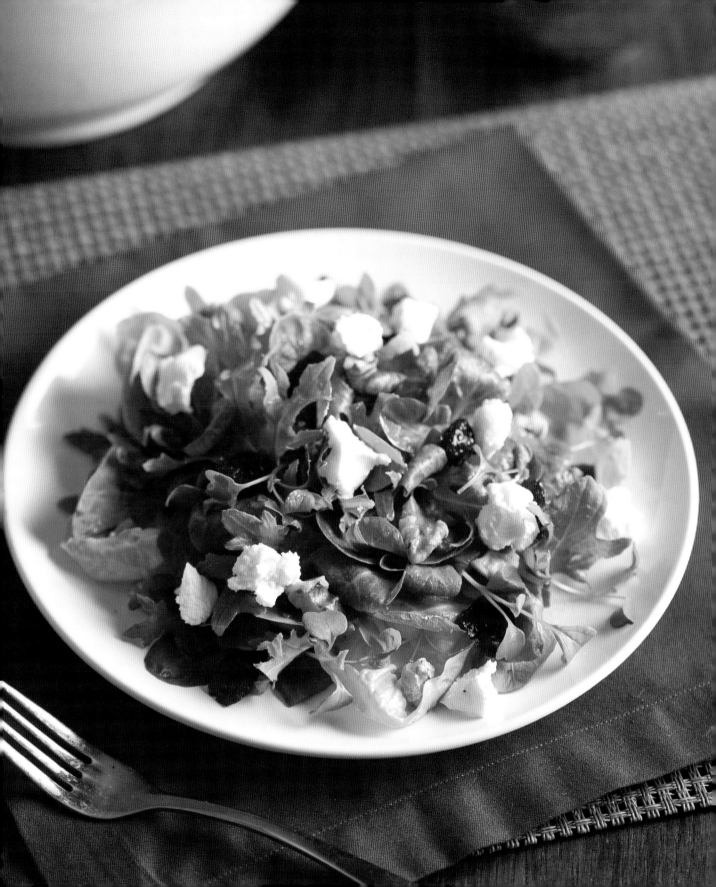

Cucumber-Jicama Salad

MAKES 6 SERVINGS

NUTRIENTS PER SERVING

CALORIES
100

TOTAL FAT
7g

SATURATED FAT
1g

CHOLESTEROL
0mg

SODIUM
100mg

CARBOHYDRATE
10g

DIETARY FIBER
4g

PROTEIN
1g

1 cucumber, unpeeled
1 jicama (1 pound)
½ cup thinly sliced red onion
2 tablespoons fresh lime juice
½ teaspoon grated lime peel
1 clove garlic, minced

¼ teaspoon salt
⅛ teaspoon crumbled dried de árbol chile or red pepper flakes
3 tablespoons vegetable oil
Leaf lettuce

1 Cut cucumber lengthwise in half; scoop out and discard seeds. Cut halves crosswise into ⅛-inch-thick slices. Peel jicama. Cut lengthwise into 8 wedges; cut wedges crosswise into ⅛-inch-thick slices.

2 Combine cucumber, jicama and onion in large bowl; toss lightly to mix; set aside.

3 Combine juice, lime peel, garlic, salt and chile in small bowl. Gradually whisk in oil until well blended.

4 Pour dressing over salad; toss lightly to coat. Cover; refrigerate 1 to 2 hours to blend flavors. Serve salad in lettuce-lined salad bowl.

TIP

To add a decorative touch to cucumber slices, score the skin of a cucumber by pulling the tines of a dinner fork along the length of the cucumber. Rotate the cucumber and repeat until completely scored. Then cut the cucumber crosswise into slices.

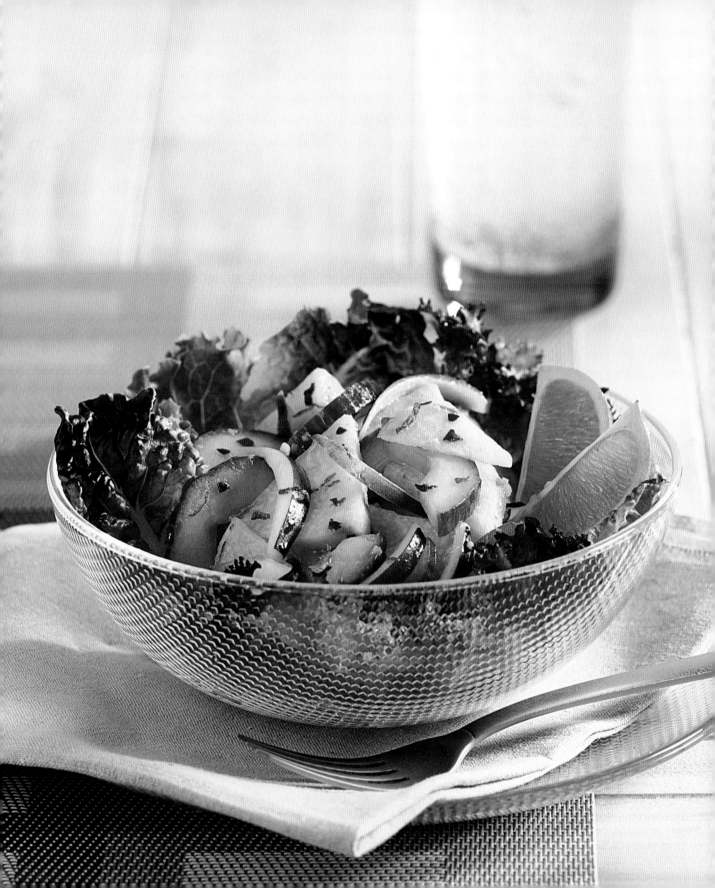

Crab Cobb Salad

MAKES 8 SERVINGS

12 cups washed and torn romaine lettuce

2 cans (6 ounces each) crabmeat, drained

2 cups diced ripe tomatoes or halved cherry tomatoes

¼ cup crumbled blue or Gorgonzola cheese

¼ cup imitation bacon bits

¾ cup fat-free or regular Italian or Caesar salad dressing

Black pepper

1 Arrange lettuce on large serving platter. Arrange crabmeat, tomatoes, blue cheese and bacon bits over lettuce.

2 Just before serving, drizzle dressing evenly over salad. Sprinkle with pepper to taste.

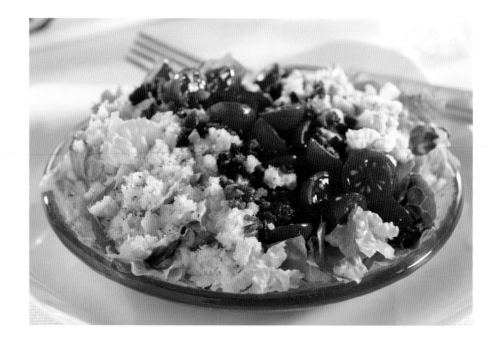

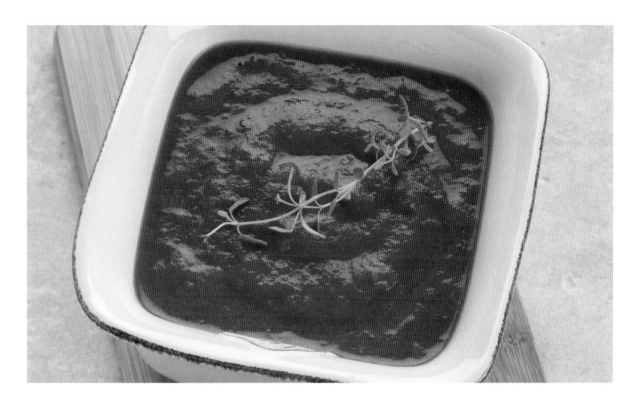

Sweet Red Bell Pepper Soup

MAKES 8 SERVINGS

NUTRIENTS PER SERVING

CALORIES
80

TOTAL FAT
4g

SATURATED FAT
1g

CHOLESTEROL
0mg

SODIUM
5mg

CARBOHYDRATE
10g

DIETARY FIBER
3g

PROTEIN
1g

- 8 red bell peppers
- 2 tablespoons olive oil
- 1 onion, thinly sliced
- 3 cloves garlic, minced
- 1 teaspoon black pepper
- 1 teaspoon dried oregano
- 2 tablespoons balsamic vinegar
- 1½ tablespoons fresh thyme, divided

SLOW COOKER DIRECTIONS

1 Cut bell peppers in half and remove stem and seeds; slice into quarters. Coat slow cooker with oil. Add bell peppers, onion, garlic, black pepper and oregano; gently mix. Cover; cook on HIGH 4 hours or until bell peppers are very tender; stirring halfway through cooking.

2 Purée soup in slow cooker using hand-held immersion blender. Or, transfer mixture in batches to blender or food processor. Blend until smooth. Stir in balsamic vinegar. Ladle soup into bowls; garnish with thyme.

Flank Steak and Roasted Vegetable Salad

NUTRIENTS PER SERVING

CALORIES
270

TOTAL FAT
11g

SATURATED FAT
3g

CHOLESTEROL
70mg

SODIUM
740mg

CARBOHYDRATE
13g

DIETARY FIBER
6g

PROTEIN
29g

MAKES 4 SERVINGS

1½ pounds asparagus spears, trimmed and cut into 2-inch lengths

½ cup baby carrots (optional)

1 tablespoon plus 1 teaspoon olive oil, divided

¾ teaspoon salt, divided

1 teaspoon black pepper, divided

1 pound flank steak (1 inch thick)

2 tablespoons plus 1 teaspoon Dijon mustard, divided

1 tablespoon fresh lemon juice

1 tablespoon water

6 cups mixed salad greens

1 Preheat oven to 400°F. Place asparagus and carrots, if desired, in shallow roasting pan. Add 1 tespoon oil, ¼ teaspoon salt and ¼ teaspoon pepper; toss to coat. Roast 20 minutes or until vegetables are browned and tender, stirring once.

2 Meanwhile, sprinkle steak with ¼ teaspoon salt and ½ teaspoon pepper. Rub both sides of steak with 2 tablespoons mustard. Place steak on rack in baking pan. Roast 10 minutes for medium-rare or to desired doneness, turning once. Let stand 5 minutes; cut across the grain into thin slices.

3 Whisk lemon juice, remaining 1 tablespoon oil, water, remaining 1 teaspoon mustard, ¼ teaspoon salt and ¼ teaspoon pepper in large bowl. Drizzle 1 tablespoon dressing over vegetables in the pan; toss to coat. Add greens to dressing in the bowl; toss to coat. Divide greens among serving plates. Top evenly with steak and vegetables.

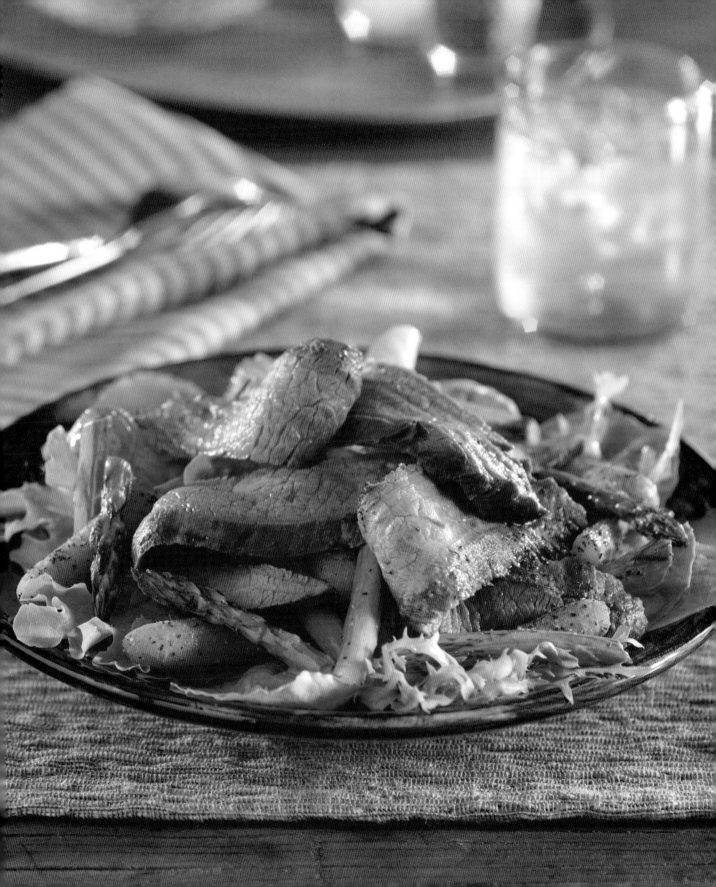

Tex-Mex Chili

MAKES 6 SERVINGS

- 4 slices bacon, diced
- 2 pounds boneless beef top round or chuck shoulder steak, trimmed and cut into ½-inch cubes
- 1 medium onion, chopped
- 2 cloves garlic, minced
- ¼ cup chili powder
- 1 teaspoon dried oregano
- 1 teaspoon ground cumin
- 1 teaspoon salt
- ½ to 1 teaspoon ground red pepper
- ½ teaspoon hot pepper sauce
- 4 cups water
- Additional chopped onion (optional)

1 Cook bacon in 5-quart Dutch oven over medium-high heat until crisp. Remove with slotted spoon; drain on paper towels.

2 Add half of beef to bacon drippings in Dutch oven; cook and stir until lightly browned. Remove beef to plate; repeat with remaining beef.

3 Add 1 chopped onion and garlic to Dutch oven; cook and stir over medium heat until onion is tender. Return beef and bacon to Dutch oven. Stir in chili powder, oregano, cumin, salt, ground red pepper, hot pepper sauce and water; bring to a boil over high heat.

4 Reduce heat to low; cover and simmer 1½ hours. Skim fat from surface; simmer, uncovered, 30 minutes or until beef is very tender and chili has thickened slightly. Garnish with additional chopped onion.

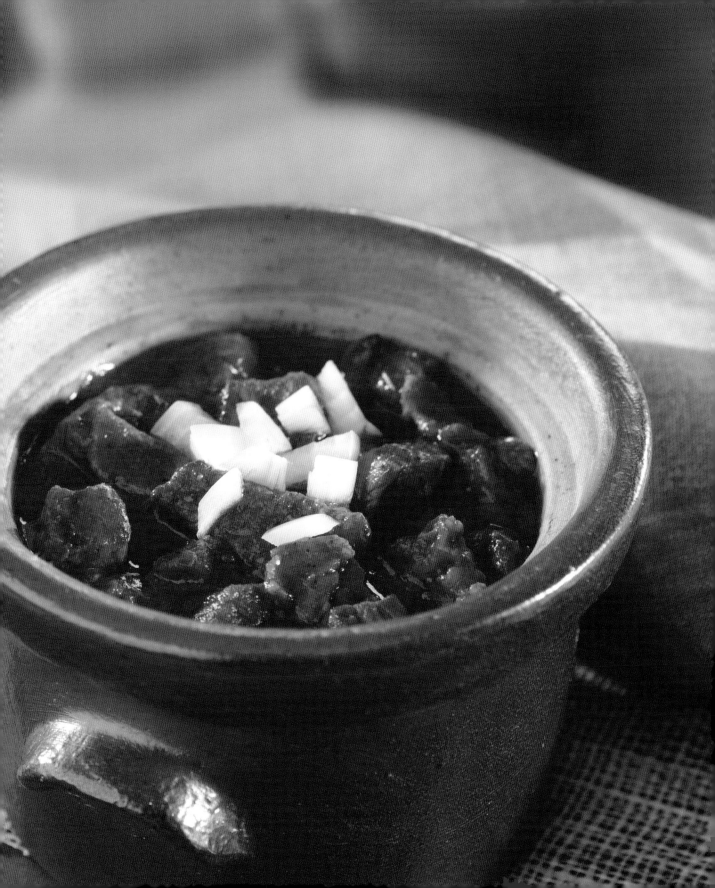

Marinated Tomato Salad

MAKES 8 SERVINGS

NUTRIENTS
PER SERVING

CALORIES
72

TOTAL FAT
4g

SATURATED FAT
1g

CHOLESTEROL
0mg

SODIUM
163mg

CARBOHYDRATE
9g

DIETARY FIBER
2g

PROTEIN
2g

1½ cups white wine or tarragon vinegar

½ teaspoon salt

¼ cup finely chopped shallots

2 tablespoons finely chopped chives

2 tablespoons fresh lemon juice

¼ teaspoon white pepper

2 tablespoons extra virgin olive oil

6 plum tomatoes, quartered

2 large yellow tomatoes,* sliced horizontally into ½-inch-thick slices

16 red cherry tomatoes, halved

16 small yellow pear tomatoes,* halved (optional)

Sunflower sprouts (optional)

Substitute 10 plum tomatoes, quartered, for yellow tomatoes and yellow pear tomatoes, if desired.

1 Combine vinegar and salt in large bowl; stir until salt is completely dissolved. Add shallots, chives, lemon juice and pepper; mix well. Gradually whisk in oil until well blended.

2 Add tomatoes to marinade; toss well. Cover; let stand at room temperature 30 minutes or up to 2 hours before serving.

3 To serve, divide salad equally among 8 plates. Garnish with sunflower sprouts.

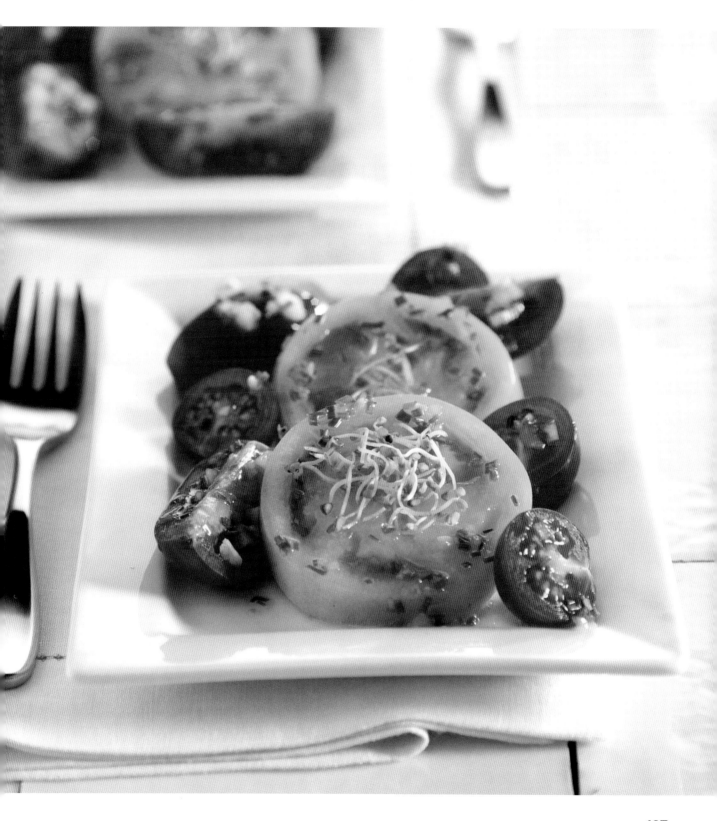

Sausage and Chicken Gumbo

MAKES 6 SERVINGS

NUTRIENTS
PER SERVING

CALORIES
239

TOTAL FAT
11g

SATURATED FAT
2g

CHOLESTEROL
103mg

SODIUM
1000mg

CARBOHYDRATE
10g

DIETARY FIBER
2g

PROTEIN
28g

1 tablespoon canola oil

1 red bell pepper, chopped

1 pound boneless skinless chicken thighs, trimmed and cut into 1-inch pieces

1 package (12 ounces) Cajun andouille or spicy chicken sausage, sliced ½ inch thick

½ cup chicken broth

1 can (28 ounces) crushed tomatoes with roasted garlic

¼ cup finely chopped green onions

1 bay leaf

½ teaspoon dried basil

½ teaspoon black pepper

¼ to ½ teaspoon red pepper flakes

6 lemon wedges (optional)

1 Heat oil in large saucepan over medium-high heat. Add bell pepper; cook and stir 2 to 3 minutes. Add chicken; cook and stir about 2 minutes or until browned. Add sausage; cook and stir 2 minutes or until browned. Add broth; scrape up browned bits from bottom of saucepan.

2 Add tomatoes, green onions, bay leaf, basil, black pepper and red pepper flakes. Simmer 15 minutes. Remove and discard bay leaf. Garnish each serving with lemon wedge, if desired.

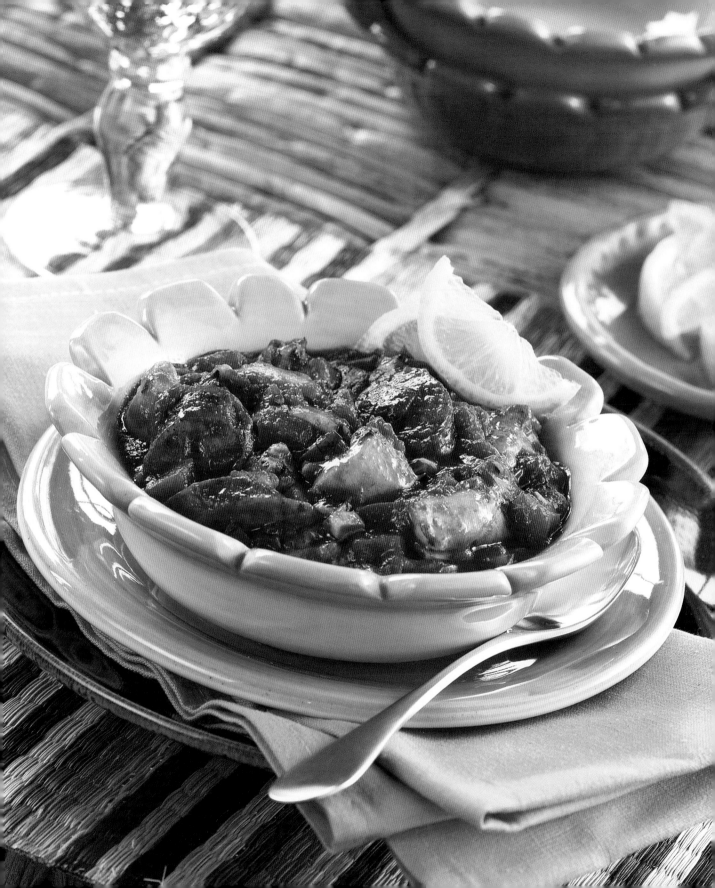

Market Salad

MAKES 4 SERVINGS

3 eggs

4 cups mixed baby salad greens

2 cups green beans, cut into 1½ inch pieces, cooked and drained

4 slices thick-cut bacon, crisp-cooked and crumbled

1 tablespoon minced fresh basil, chiles, or Italian parsley

3 tablespoons olive oil

1 tablespoon red wine vinegar

1 teaspoon Dijon mustard

¼ teaspoon salt

¼ teaspoon black pepper

1 Place eggs in small saucepan with enough water to cover; bring to a boil over medium-high heat. Immediately remove from heat. Cover; let stand 10 minutes. Drain; cool eggs to room temperature.

2 Combine salad greens, green beans, bacon and basil in large serving bowl. Peel and coarsely chop eggs; add to serving bowl. Whisk oil, vinegar, mustard, salt and pepper in small bowl until well blended. Drizzle dressing over salad; toss gently to coat.

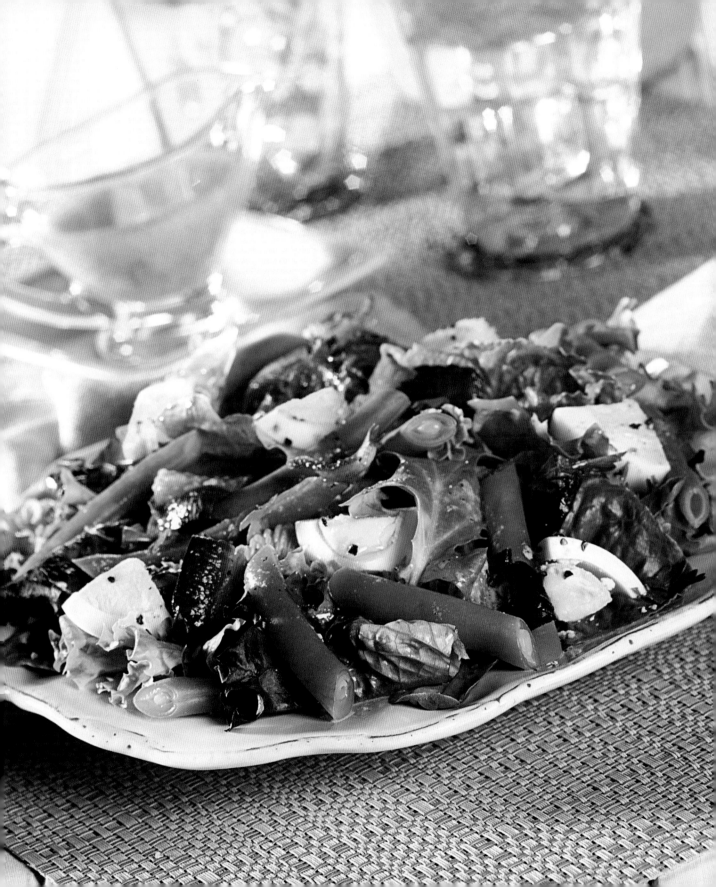

Spring Greens with Blueberries, Walnuts and Feta Cheese

NUTRIENTS PER SERVING

CALORIES
146

TOTAL FAT
11g

SATURATED FAT
2g

CHOLESTEROL
5mg

SODIUM
300mg

CARBOHYDRATE
8g

DIETARY FIBER
3g

PROTEIN
5g

MAKES 4 SERVINGS

1 tablespoon canola oil

1 tablespoon white wine vinegar or sherry vinegar

2 teaspoons Dijon mustard

½ teaspoon salt (optional)

½ teaspoon black pepper

5 cups mixed spring greens (5 ounces)

1 cup fresh blueberries

½ cup reduced-fat or regular crumbled feta cheese

¼ cup chopped walnuts or pecans, toasted*

To toast nuts, place in nonstick skillet. Cook and stir over medium-low heat until nuts begin to brown, about 5 minutes. Remove immediately to plate to cool.

1 Whisk oil, vinegar, mustard, salt, if desired, and pepper in large bowl.

2 Add greens and blueberries; toss gently to coat. Top with cheese and walnuts. Serve immediately.

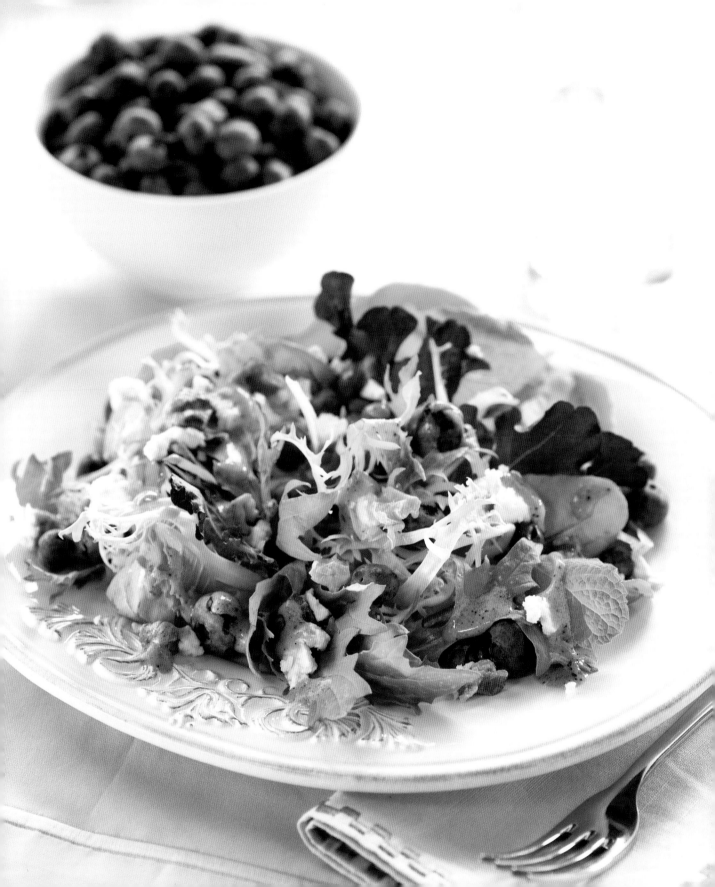

BEEF, PORK AND LAMB

Steak Parmesan

MAKES 3 SERVINGS

4 cloves garlic, minced
¾ teaspoon olive oil
1 tablespoon coarse salt
1 teaspoon dried rosemary

1 teaspoon black pepper
2 beef T-bone or Porterhouse steaks, cut 1 inch thick (about 2 pounds)
¼ cup grated Parmesan cheese

1 Prepare grill for direct cooking. Combine garlic, oil, salt, rosemary and pepper in small bowl; press into both sides of steaks. Let stand 15 minutes.

2 Place steaks on grid over medium-high heat. Cover; grill 14 to 19 minutes or until internal temperature reaches 145°F for medium-rare doneness, turning once.

3 Transfer steaks to cutting board; sprinkle with cheese. Tent with foil; let stand 5 minutes. Serve immediately.

TIP

For a smoky flavor, soak 2 cups hickory or oak wood chips in cold water to cover at least 30 minutes. Drain and scatter over hot coals before grilling. Makes 2 to 3 servings.

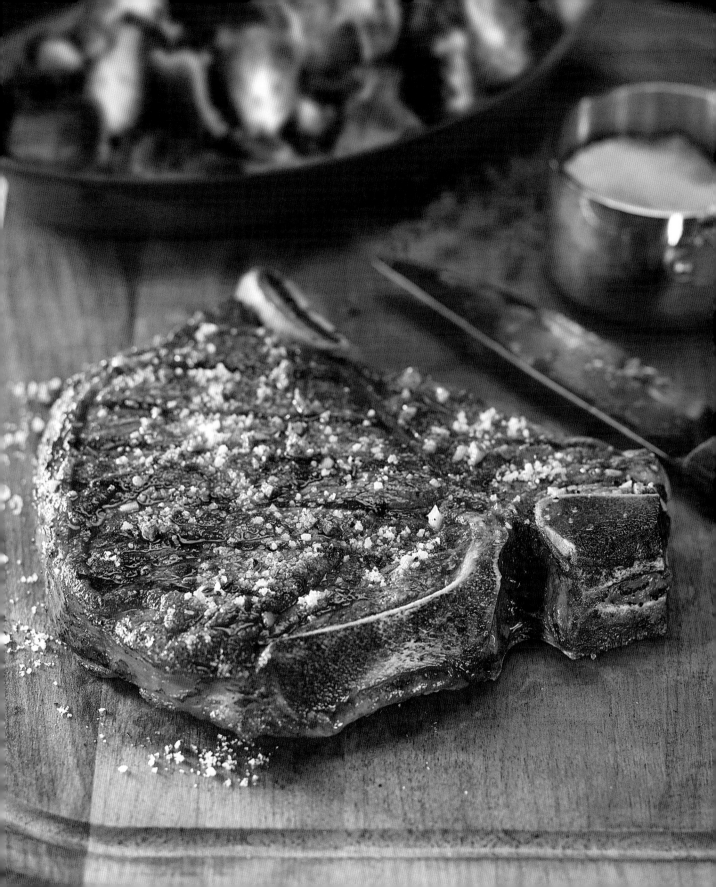

Pork with Cucumber Pico de Gallo

MAKES 4 SERVINGS (3 OUNCES PORK AND ¼ CUP CUCUMBER MIXTURE PER SERVING)

½ medium unpeeled cucumber, seeded and finely chopped (4 ounces total)

2 medium tomatillos, husks removed, rinsed and chopped

2 tablespoons chopped fresh cilantro

⅛ teaspoon red pepper flakes

1 to 2 tablespoons lime juice

¼ teaspoon salt, divided

4 boneless center-cut pork cutlets, trimmed of fat (about 1 pound)

¼ teaspoon coarsely ground black pepper

Nonstick cooking spray *or* 2 teaspoons olive oil

1 Combine cucumber, tomatillos, cilantro, red pepper flakes, lime juice, and ⅛ teaspoon salt in a mixing bowl. Toss gently to blend. Set aside.

2 Coat pork chops evenly with black pepper and remaining ⅛ teaspoon salt.

3 Spray large nonstick skillet with cooking spray or place oil in skillet; heat over medium-high heat. Add pork; immediately reduce heat to medium. Cook 5 minutes. Turn and cook 4 to 5 minutes longer or until barely pink in center. Serve with cucumber mixture.

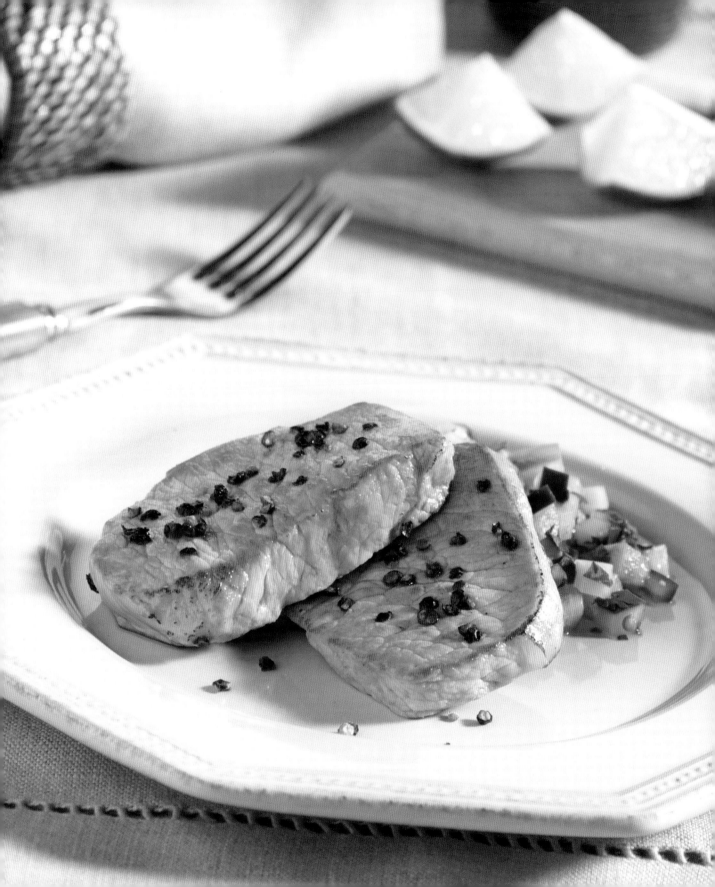

Skirt Steak with Red Pepper Chimichurri

MAKES 4 SERVINGS

- 1 pound skirt steak, trimmed
- 1 clove garlic, peeled and cut in half
- ¼ teaspoon salt
- ½ teaspoon black pepper, divided
- 1 cup diced roasted red bell pepper
- 1 shallot, minced
- 1 tablespoon capers
- 1½ tablespoons olive oil
- 1 tablespoon white wine vinegar
- 1 clove garlic, minced

1 Preheat broiler. Spray broiler rack with nonstick cooking spray. Rub garlic clove over both sides of steak. Season with salt and ¼ teaspoon black pepper. Place steak on broiler rack. Broil steak, 4 inches from heat, 4 to 5 minutes per side or until desired doneness.

2 To prepare chimichurri sauce, combine red bell pepper, shallot, capers, oil, vinegar, minced garlic and remaining ¼ teaspoon black pepper in a bowl.

3 To serve, thinly slice skirt steak against the grain and arrange on a serving platter. Top with chimichurri sauce.

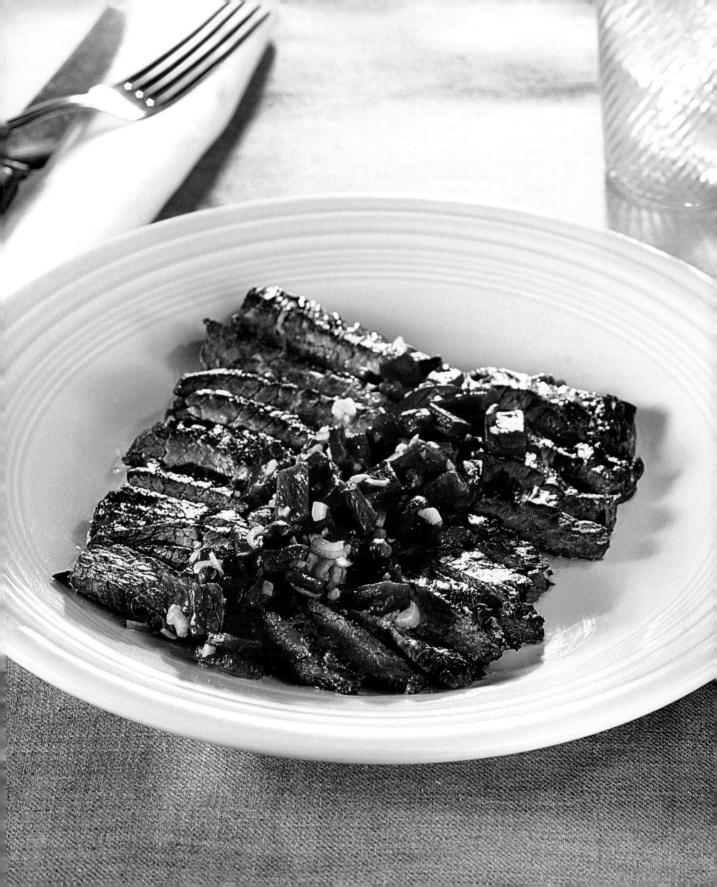

Pork Tenderloin with Avocado-Tomatillo Salsa

MAKES 4 SERVINGS (3 OUNCES PORK AND ¼ CUP SALSA PER SERVING)

NUTRIENTS PER SERVING

CALORIES
174

TOTAL FAT
6g

SATURATED FAT
1g

CHOLESTEROL
73mg

SODIUM
278mg

CARBOHYDRATE
4g

DIETARY FIBER
2g

PROTEIN
25g

1½ teaspoons chili powder

½ teaspoon ground cumin

1 pound pork tenderloin

1 teaspoon extra virgin olive oil

SALSA

2 medium tomatillos, husked and diced*

½ ripe medium avocado, diced

1 jalapeño pepper, seeded and finely chopped

1 clove garlic, minced

2 tablespoons finely chopped red onion

1 tablespoon lime juice

1 to 2 tablespoons chopped fresh cilantro

⅛ teaspoon salt

4 lime wedges (optional)

Remove the husk by pulling from the bottom to where it attaches at the stem, Wash before using.

1 Preheat oven to 425°F. Combine chili powder and cumin in small bowl; sprinkle all over pork and press to adhere.

2 Heat oil in large nonstick skillet over medium-high heat. Add pork; cook 3 minutes. Turn; cook 2 to 3 minutes longer or until well browned. Place on foil-lined baking sheet; bake 20 to 25 minutes or until barely pink in center (about 165°F). Remove from oven and let stand 5 minutes before slicing.

3 Combine tomatillos, avocado, jalapeño, garlic, onion, lime juice, cilantro and salt in small bowl; toss gently to blend. Serve with pork slices and lime wedges, if desired.

TIP

Choose firm tomatillos with dry husks that are not too ragged. Store in a paper bag in refrigerator for up to a month.

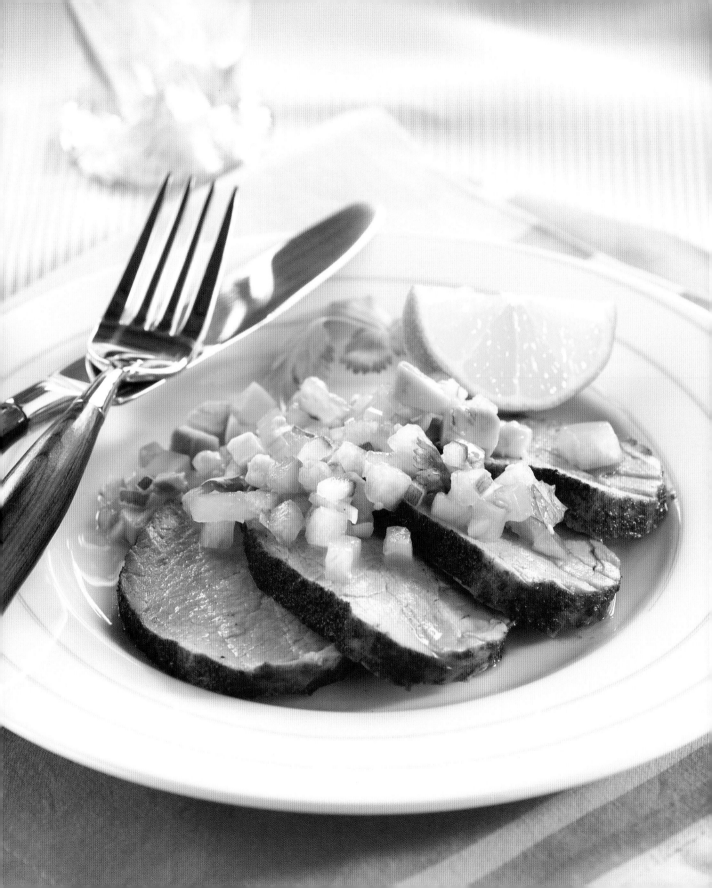

Pork Roast with Dijon Tarragon Glaze

MAKES 4 TO 6 SERVINGS

NUTRIENTS PER SERVING

CALORIES
170

TOTAL FAT
6g

SATURATED FAT
2g

CHOLESTEROL
73mg

SODIUM
189mg

CARBOHYDRATE
2g

DIETARY FIBER
1g

PROTEIN
25g

2 tablespoons Dijon mustard

1 teaspoon minced fresh tarragon

2 tablespoons lemon juice

⅓ cup reduced-sodium chicken or vegetable broth

1½ to 2 pounds boneless pork loin, trimmed

½ teaspoon freshly ground black pepper

1 teaspoon ground paprika

1 Preheat oven to 350°F. For glaze, combine mustard, tarragon, lemon juice and broth in small bowl; set aside.

2 Line roasting pan with foil. Place pork on rack in prepared pan. Sprinkle roast with pepper and paprika. Bake 15 minutes. Remove roast from oven. Spoon glaze evenly over roast; bake 20 minutes. Baste roast with pan drippings. Bake 20 to 30 minutes or until internal temperature reaches 160°F.

3 Remove roast from oven; let stand 15 minutes before slicing.

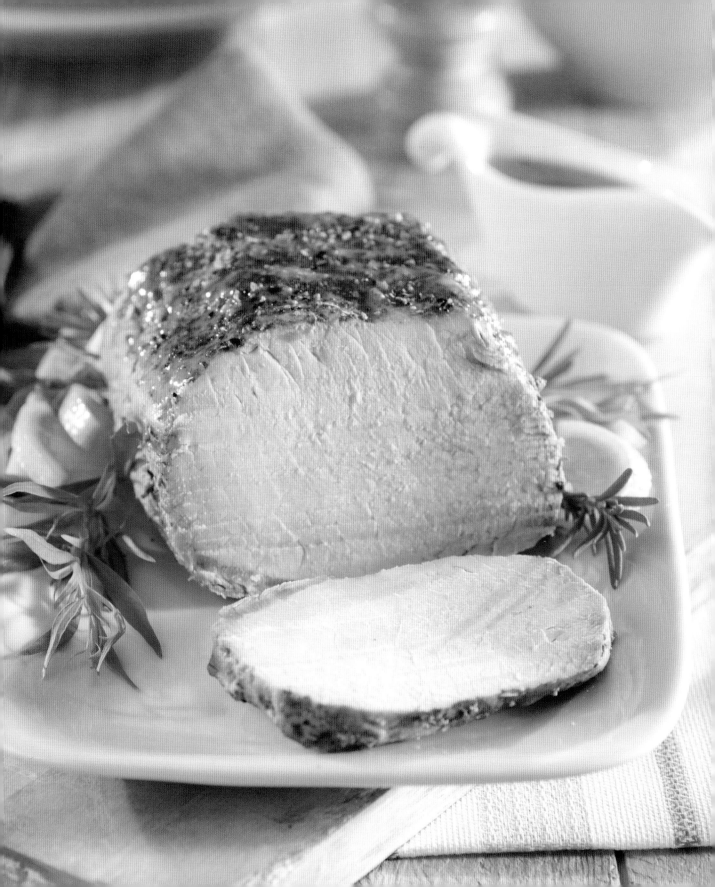

Herbed Standing Rib Roast

MAKES 16 (6-OUNCE) SERVINGS

- 2 teaspoons kosher salt
- 1 (4-rib) bone-in standing rib roast (about 9 pounds)
- 2 tablespoons olive oil
- 4 cloves garlic, minced
- 2 teaspoons grated lemon peel
- 2 tablespoons chopped fresh rosemary
- 2 tablespoons chopped fresh thyme
- 2 tablespoons chopped fresh Italian parsley
- 2 tablespoons chopped fresh oregano
- 2 teaspoons black pepper
- ¼ teaspoon red pepper flakes

1 Sprinkle salt over entire roast. Wrap with plastic wrap and refrigerate at least 2 hours or up to 2 days.

2 Combine oil, garlic, lemon peel, rosemary, thyme, parsley, oregano, black pepper and red pepper flakes in small bowl; mix well. Rub paste all over roast. Allow roast to sit at room temperature at least 1 hour or up to 2 hours.

3 Preheat oven to 450°F. Spray roasting pan just large enough to fit roast with nonstick cooking spray. Place roast, bone side down, in prepared pan. Roast 25 minutes. *Reduce oven temperature to 350°F.* Roast 1½ to 2 hours or until meat thermometer inserted into thickest part of roast registers 120° to 125°F (rare), or 130° to 140°F (medium-rare). Tent with foil. Let stand 15 to 20 minutes before slicing.

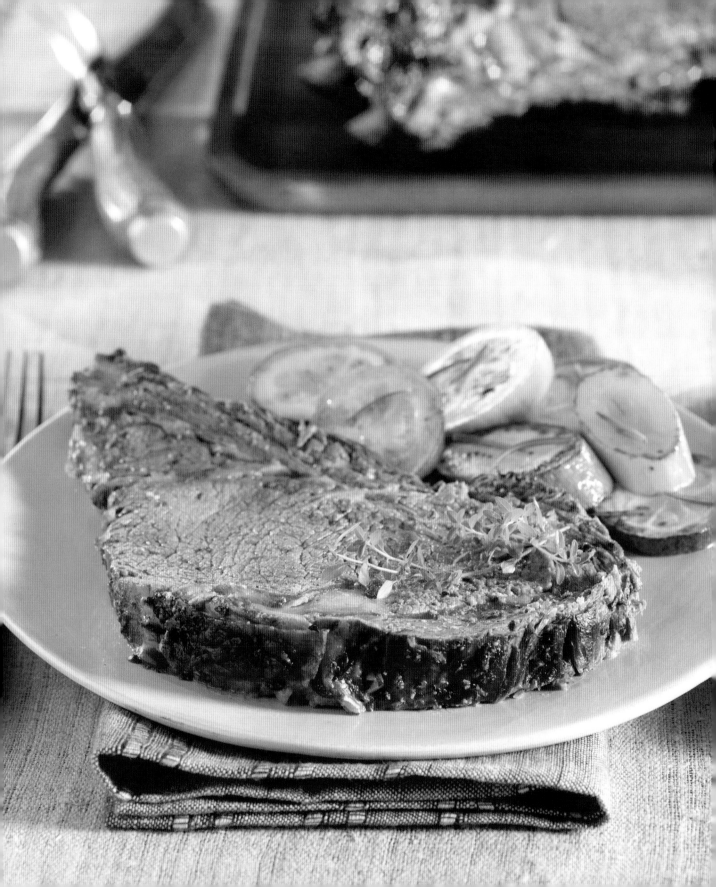

Greek Lamb with Tzatziki Sauce

MAKES 4 SERVINGS

2½ to 3 pounds boneless leg of lamb

8 cloves garlic, divided

¼ cup Dijon mustard

2 tablespoons minced fresh rosemary leaves

2 teaspoons salt

2 teaspoons black pepper

¼ cup plus 2 teaspoons olive oil, divided

1 small seedless cucumber

1 tablespoon chopped fresh mint

1 teaspoon lemon juice

2 cups plain nonfat or regular Greek yogurt

1 Untie and unroll lamb to lie flat; trim fat.

2 For marinade, mince 4 garlic cloves; place in small bowl. Add mustard, rosemary, salt and pepper; whisk in ¼ cup oil. Spread mixture evenly over lamb, coating both sides. Place lamb in large resealable food storage bag. Seal bag; refrigerate at least 2 hours or overnight, turning several times.

3 Meanwhile for tzatziki sauce, mince remaining 4 garlic cloves and mash to a paste; place in medium bowl. Peel and grate cucumber; squeeze to remove excess moisture. Add cucumber, mint, remaining 2 teaspoons oil and lemon juice to bowl with garlic. Add yogurt; mix well. Refrigerate until ready to serve.

4 Prepare grill for direct cooking. Grill lamb over medium-high heat 35 to 40 minutes or to desired doneness. Cover loosely with foil; let rest 5 to 10 minutes. (Remove from grill at 140°F for medium. Temperature will rise 5°F while resting.)

5 Slice lamb and serve with tzatziki sauce.

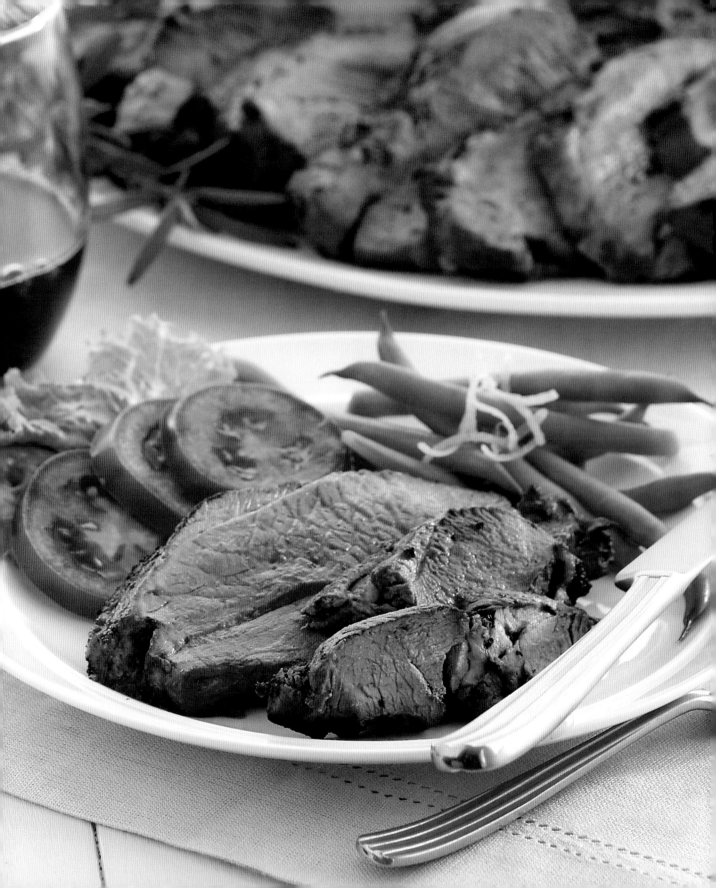

Sesame-Garlic Flank Steak

MAKES 4 SERVINGS

NUTRIENTS PER SERVING

CALORIES
250

TOTAL FAT
11g

SATURATED FAT
4g

CHOLESTEROL
90mg

SODIUM
790mg

CARBOHYDRATE
5g

DIETARY FIBER
0g

PROTEIN
31g

1 flank steak (about 1¼ pounds)
2 tablespoons soy sauce
2 tablespoons hoisin sauce
1 tablespoon dark sesame oil
2 cloves garlic, minced

1 Score steak lightly with sharp knife in diamond pattern on both sides; place in large resealable food storage bag. Combine soy sauce, hoisin sauce, sesame oil and garlic in small bowl; pour over steak. Seal bag; turn to coat. Marinate in refrigerator at least 2 hours or up to 24 hours, turning once.

2 Prepare grill for direct cooking. Remove steak from marinade; reserve marinade. Grill steak, covered, over medium heat 13 to 18 minutes for medium rare (145°F) to medium (160°F) or to desired doneness, turning and brushing with marinade halfway through cooking time. Discard remaining marinade.

3 Transfer steak to cutting board; carve across the grain into thin slices.

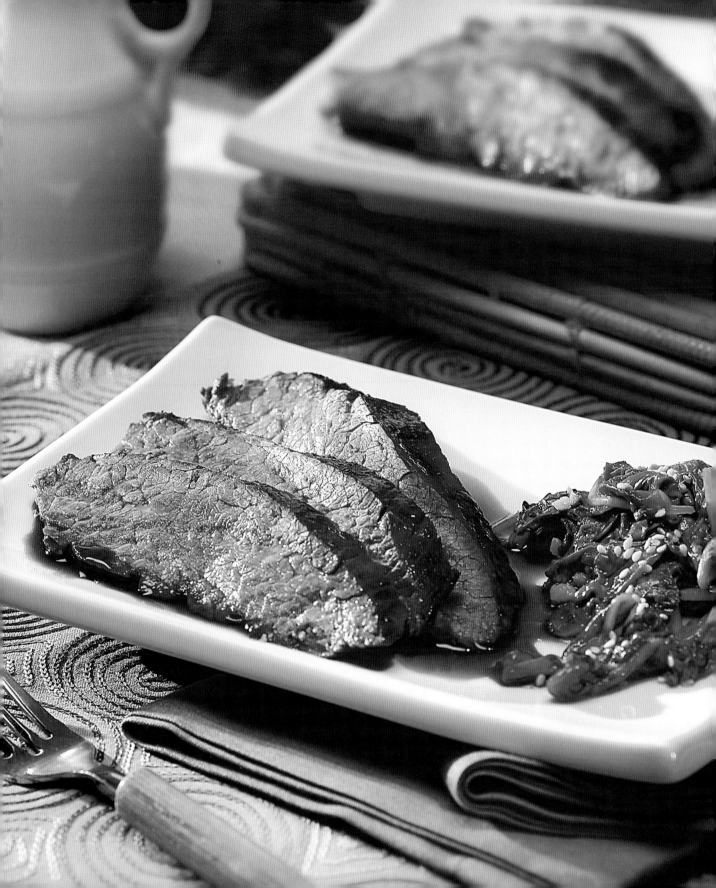

Steak Fajitas

MAKES 4 SERVINGS

¼ cup lime juice

2 tablespoons soy sauce

4 tablespoons vegetable oil, divided

2 tablespoons Worcestershire sauce

2 cloves garlic, minced

½ teaspoon ground red pepper

1 pound flank steak, skirt steak or top sirloin

1 small yellow onion, halved and cut into ¼-inch slices

1 green bell pepper, cut into ¼-inch strips

1 red bell pepper, cut into ¼-inch strips

Lime wedges (optional)

Pico de gallo, guacamole, sour cream, shredded lettuce and shredded Cheddar-Jack cheese (optional)

1 Combine lime juice, soy sauce, 2 tablespoons oil, Worcestershire sauce, garlic and ground red pepper in medium bowl; mix well. Remove ¼ cup marinade to large bowl. Place steak in large resealable food storage bag. Pour remaining marinade over steak; seal bag and turn to coat. Marinate in refrigerator at least 2 hours or overnight. Add onion and bell peppers to bowl with ¼ cup marinade; toss to coat. Cover and refrigerate until ready to use.

2 Remove steak from marinade; discard marinade and wipe off excess from steak. Heat 1 tablespoon oil in large skillet over medium-high heat. Cook steak about 4 minutes per side for medium rare or to desired doneness. Remove to cutting board; tent with foil and let rest 10 minutes.

3 Meanwhile, heat remaining 1 tablespoon oil in same skillet over medium-high heat. Add vegetable mixture; cook about 8 minutes or until vegetables are crisp-tender and beginning to brown in spots, stirring occasionally. (Cook in 2 batches if necessary; do not pile vegetables in skillet.)

4 Cut steak into thin slices across the grain. Serve with vegetables, tortillas, lime wedges and desired toppings.

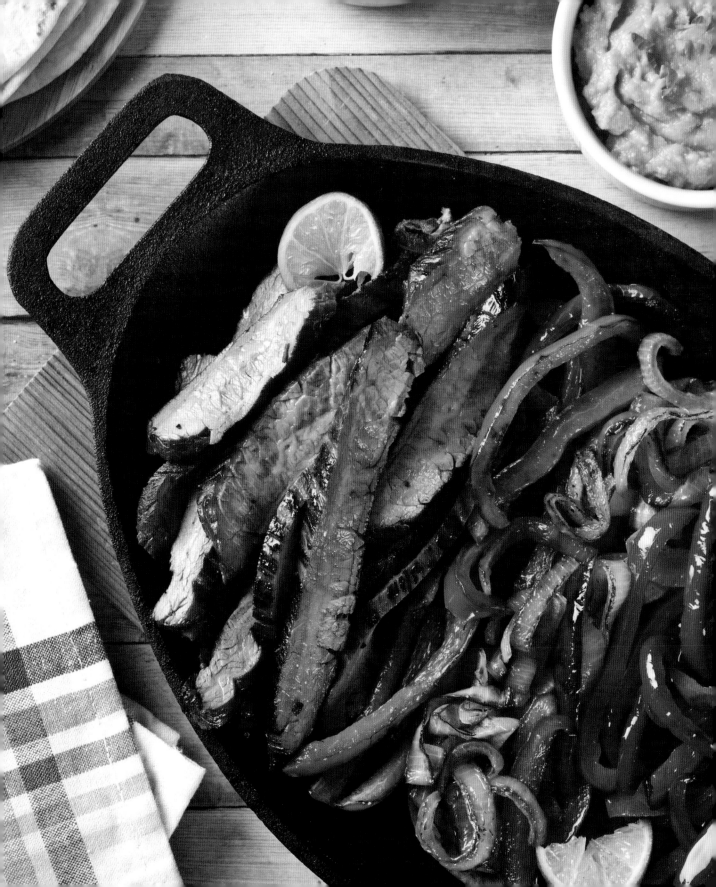

Zesty Skillet Pork Chops

MAKES 4 SERVINGS

NUTRIENTS PER SERVING

CALORIES
172

TOTAL FAT
7g

SATURATED FAT
2g

CHOLESTEROL
49mg

SODIUM
387mg

CARBOHYDRATE
9g

DIETARY FIBER
3g

PROTEIN
20g

1 teaspoon chili powder

½ teaspoon salt, divided

4 lean boneless pork chops (about 1¼ pounds), well trimmed

2 cups diced tomatoes

1 cup chopped green, red or yellow bell pepper

¾ cup thinly sliced celery

½ cup chopped onion

1 teaspoon dried thyme

1 tablespoon hot pepper sauce

Nonstick cooking spray *or* 2 teaspoons olive oil

2 tablespoons finely chopped fresh parsley

1 Rub chili powder and ¼ teaspoon salt evenly over one side of pork chops.

2 Combine tomatoes, bell pepper, celery, onion, thyme and hot pepper sauce in medium bowl; mix well.

3 Lightly spray large nonstick skillet with nonstick cooking spray or place oil in skillet; heat over medium-high heat. Add pork, seasoned side down; cook 1 minute. Turn pork. Top with tomato mixture; bring to a boil. Reduce heat to low. Cover; cook 25 minutes or until pork is tender and tomato mixture has thickened.

4 Transfer pork to serving plates. Bring tomato mixture to a boil over high heat; cook 2 minutes or until most liquid has evaporated. Remove from heat; stir in parsley and remaining ¼ teaspoon salt. Spoon sauce over pork.

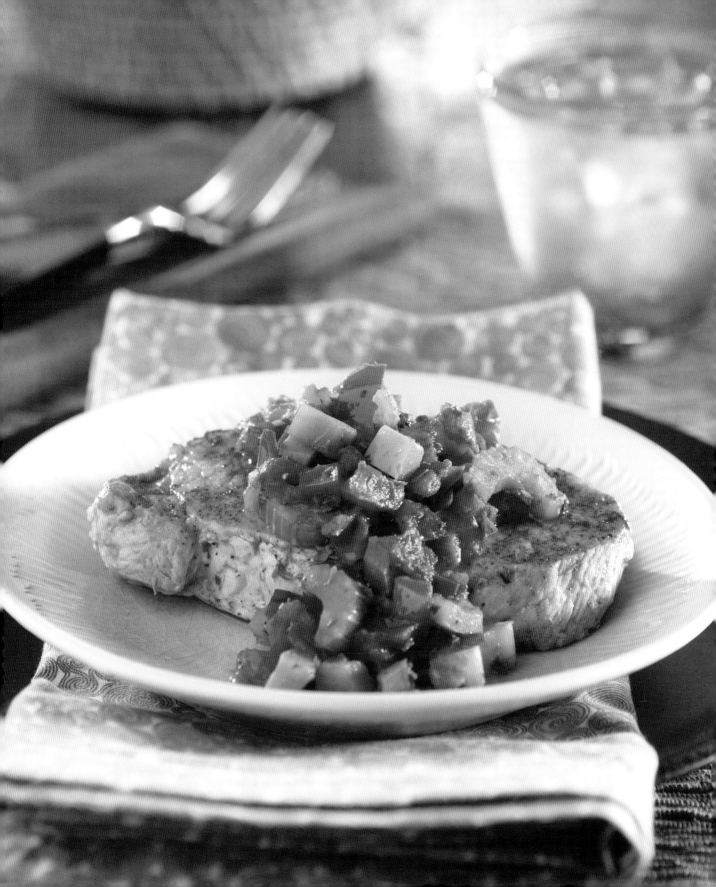

London Broil with Marinated Vegetables

MAKES 6 SERVINGS

¾ cup olive oil

¾ cup red wine

2 tablespoons finely chopped shallots

2 tablespoons red wine vinegar

2 teaspoons minced garlic

½ teaspoon dried thyme

½ teaspoon dried oregano

½ teaspoon dried basil

½ teaspoon black pepper

2 pounds top round London broil (1½ inches thick)

1 medium red onion, cut into ¼-inch-thick slices

1 package (8 ounces) sliced mushrooms

1 medium red bell pepper, cut into strips

1 medium zucchini, cut into ¼-inch-thick slices

1 Whisk oil, wine, shallots, vinegar, garlic, thyme, oregano, basil and black pepper in medium bowl until well blended. Combine London broil and ¾ cup marinade in large resealable food storage bag. Seal bag; turn to coat. Marinate in refrigerator up to 24 hours, turning bag once or twice.

2 Combine onion, mushrooms, bell pepper, zucchini and remaining marinade in separate large food storage bag. Seal bag and turn to coat. Refrigerate up to 24 hours, turning bag once or twice.

3 Preheat broiler. Remove beef from marinade and place on broiler pan; discard marinade. Broil 4 to 5 inches from heat about 9 minutes per side or until desired doneness. Let stand 10 minutes before slicing. Cut beef into thin slices.

4 Meanwhile, drain vegetables and arrange on broiler pan; discard marinade. Broil 4 to 5 inches from heat about 9 minutes or until edges of vegetables just begin to brown. Serve beef and vegetables immediately on platter.

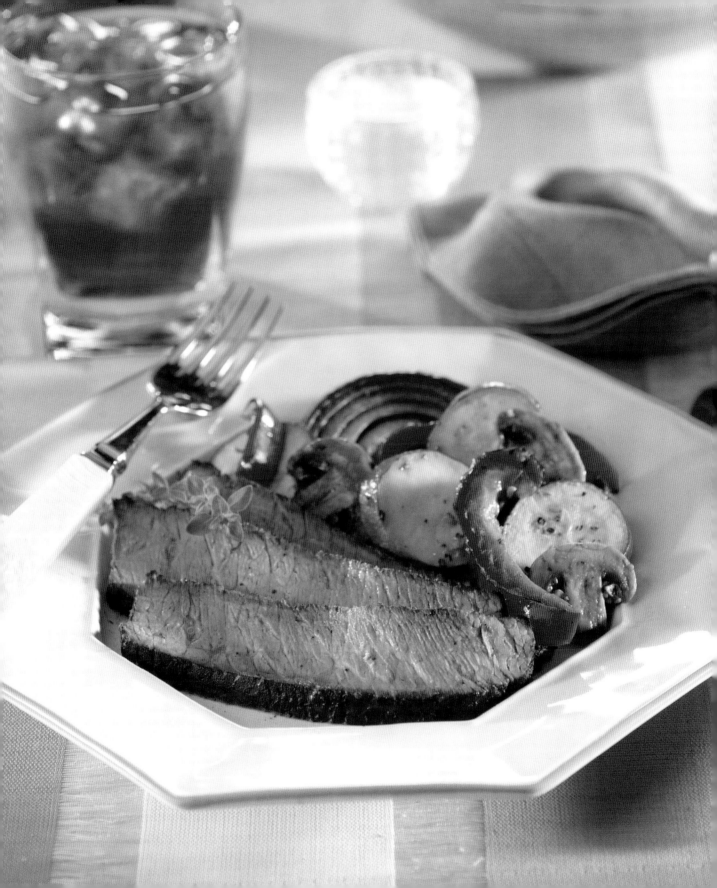

Beef Skewers

MAKES 3 SERVINGS (6 SKEWERS EACH)

NUTRIENTS
PER SERVING

CALORIES
240

TOTAL FAT
8g

SATURATED FAT
2g

CHOLESTEROL
120mg

SODIUM
198mg

CARBOHYDRATE
4g

DIETARY FIBER
2g

PROTEIN
40g

1 beef top round steak (about 1 pound)

2 tablespoons reduced-sodium soy sauce

1 tablespoon dry sherry

1 teaspoon dark sesame oil

2 cloves garlic, minced

Salt and black pepper

Mixed greens and halved cherry tomatoes (optional)

1 Cut beef crosswise into 18 (⅛-inch-thick) slices. Place in large resealable food storage bag. Combine soy sauce, sherry, oil and garlic in small cup; pour over beef. Seal bag; turn to coat. Marinate in refrigerator at least 30 minutes or up to 2 hours.

2 Meanwhile, soak 18 (6-inch) wooden skewers in water 20 minutes.

3 Preheat broiler. Drain beef; discard marinade. Weave beef accordion-style onto skewers. Place on rack of broiler pan.

4 Broil 4 to 5 inches from heat 2 minutes. Turn skewers over; broil 2 minutes more or until beef is barely pink. Season with salt and pepper, if desired. Serve warm on a bed of mixed greens and tomatoes, if desired.

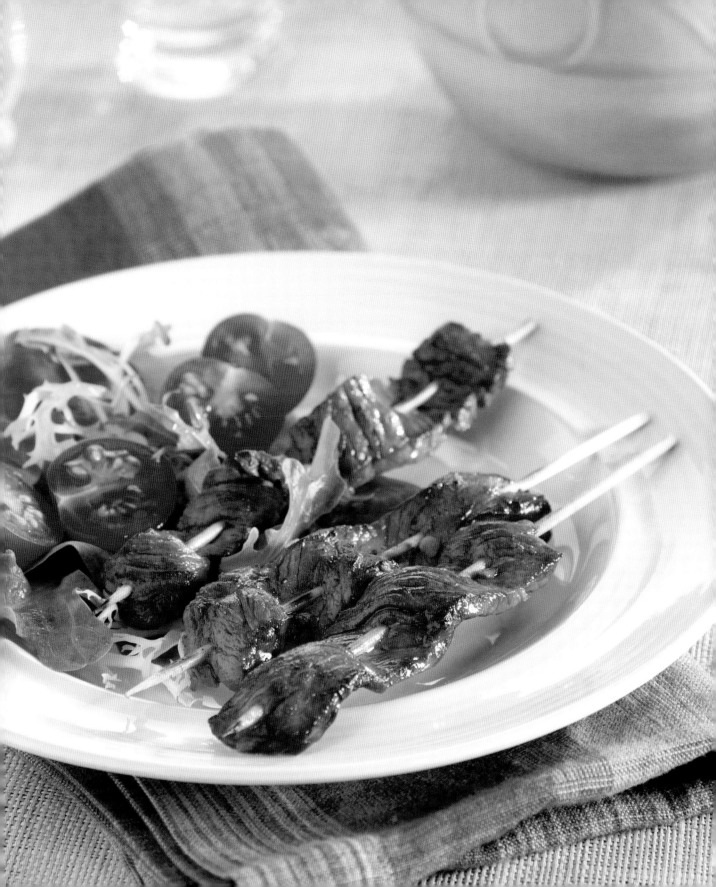

Korean Beef Short Ribs

MAKES 6 SERVINGS

NUTRIENTS PER SERVING

CALORIES
170

TOTAL FAT
11g

SATURATED FAT
4g

CHOLESTEROL
45mg

SODIUM
810mg

CARBOHYDRATE
2g

DIETARY FIBER
0g

PROTEIN
16g

2½ pounds beef chuck flanken-style short ribs, cut ⅜ to ½ inch thick*

¼ cup chopped green onions

¼ cup water

¼ cup soy sauce

2 teaspoons grated fresh ginger

2 teaspoons dark sesame oil

2 cloves garlic, minced

½ teaspoon black pepper

1 tablespoon sesame seeds, toasted

Flanken-style ribs can be ordered from your butcher. They are cross-cut short ribs sawed through the bones.

1 Place ribs in large resealable food storage bag. Combine green onions, water, soy sauce, ginger, oil, garlic and pepper in small bowl; pour over ribs. Seal bag; turn to coat. Marinate in refrigerator at least 4 hours or up to 8 hours, turning occasionally.

2 Prepare grill for direct cooking. Remove ribs from marinade; reserve marinade. Grill ribs, covered, over medium-high heat 5 minutes. Brush lightly with reserved marinade; turn and brush again. Discard remaining marinade. Continue to grill, covered, 5 to 6 minutes for medium or to desired doneness. Sprinkle with sesame seeds.

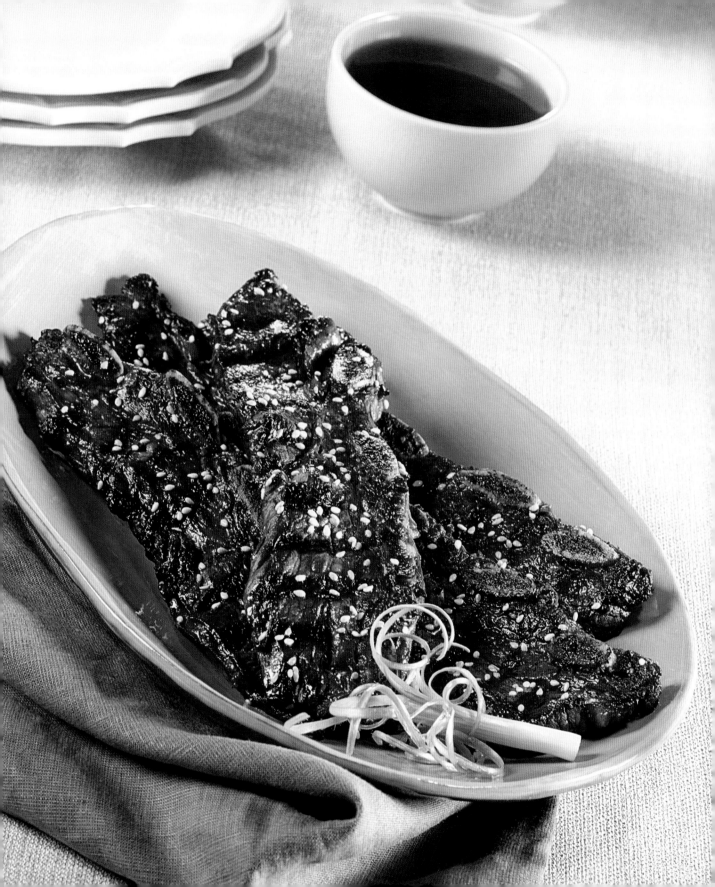

Tomato and Red Wine Brisket

MAKES 8 SERVINGS

NUTRIENTS PER SERVING

CALORIES
370

TOTAL FAT
18g

SATURATED FAT
7g

CHOLESTEROL
135mg

SODIUM
390mg

CARBOHYDRATE
7g

DIETARY FIBER
2g

PROTEIN
42g

1 beef brisket (3 to 3½ pounds), trimmed*

¾ teaspoon salt, divided

¼ teaspoon black pepper

1 tablespoon olive oil

1 large red onion, sliced

½ cup dry red wine

1 can (28 ounces) diced tomatoes with basil, oregano and garlic

If your slow cookier is less than 5 quarts, cut roast in half so it cooks completely.

SLOW COOKER DIRECTIONS

1 Coat inside of slow cooker with nonstick cooking spray. Season beef with ½ teaspoon salt and pepper. Heat oil in large skillet over medium-high heat. Add beef; cook 5 minutes per side until browned. Remove to slow cooker.

2 Return skillet to medium-high heat. Add onion; cook and stir 5 minutes or until softened. Pour in wine. Bring mixture to a boil, scraping up any browned bits from bottom of skillet. Cook 3 to 4 minutes until mixture nearly evaporates. Stir in tomatoes. Bring to a boil; cook 6 to 7 minutes or until slightly thickened. Stir in remaining ¼ teaspoon salt. Pour mixture over beef in slow cooker.

3 Cover; cook on LOW 7 to 8 hours. Remove beef to large cutting board; cover loosely with foil. Let stand 15 minutes before slicing. Turn slow cooker to HIGH. Cook, uncovered, on HIGH 10 minutes or until sauce is thickened. Serve sauce over brisket.

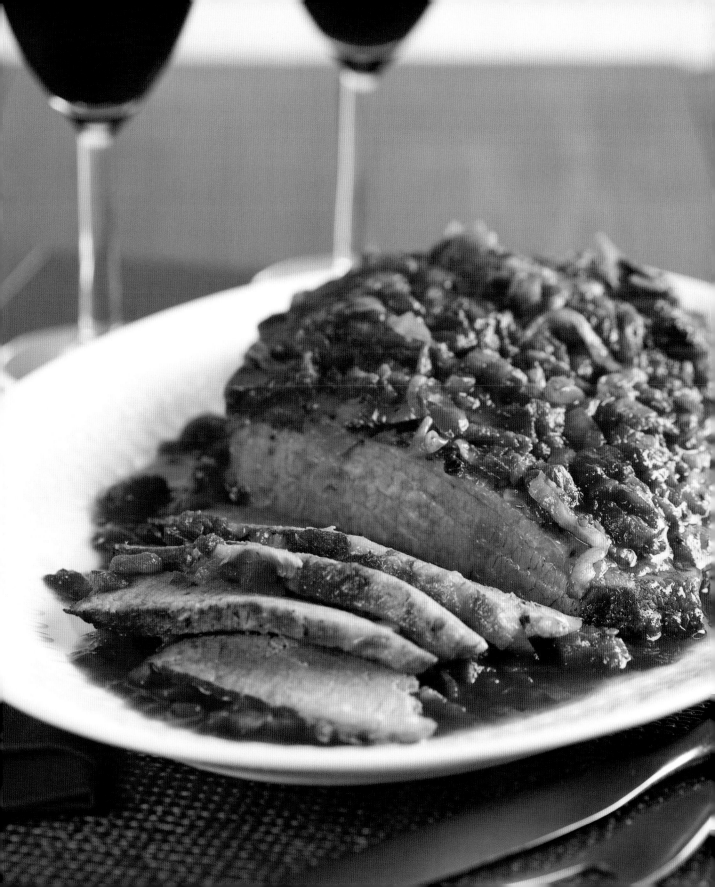

French Quarter Steaks

MAKES 2 SERVINGS

- ½ cup water
- 2 tablespoons Worcestershire sauce
- 2 tablespoons soy sauce
- 1 tablespoon chili powder
- 3 cloves garlic, minced, divided
- 2 teaspoons paprika
- 1½ teaspoons ground red pepper
- 1¼ teaspoons black pepper, divided
- 1 teaspoon onion powder
- 2 top sirloin steaks (about 8 ounces each, 1 inch thick)
- 3 tablespoons butter, divided
- 1 tablespoon olive oil
- ½ large onion, thinly sliced
- 8 ounces sliced white or shiitake mushrooms or a combination
- ¼ teaspoon plus ⅛ teaspoon salt, divided

1 Combine water, Worcestershire sauce, soy sauce, chili powder, 2 cloves garlic, paprika, red pepper, 1 teaspoon black pepper and onion powder in small bowl; mix well. Place steaks in large resealable food storage bag; pour marinade over steaks. Seal bag; turn to coat. Marinate in refrigerator 1 to 3 hours.

2 Remove steaks from marinade 30 minutes before cooking; discard marinade and pat steaks dry with paper towel. Prepare grill for direct cooking. Oil grid.

3 While grill is preheating, heat 1 tablespoon butter and 1 tablespoon oil in large skillet over medium high heat. Add onion; cook 5 minutes, stirring occasionally. Add mushrooms, ¼ teaspoon salt and remaining ¼ teaspoon black pepper; cook 10 minutes or until onion is golden brown and mushrooms are beginning to brown, stirring occasionally. Combine remaining 2 tablespoons butter, 1 clove garlic and ⅛ teaspoon salt in small skillet; cook over medium-low heat 3 minutes or until garlic begins to sizzle.

4 Grill steaks over medium-high heat 6 minutes; turn and grill 6 minutes for medium rare or until desired doneness. Brush both sides of steaks with garlic butter during last 2 minutes of cooking. Remove to plate and tent with foil; let rest 5 minutes. Serve steaks with onion and mushroom mixture.

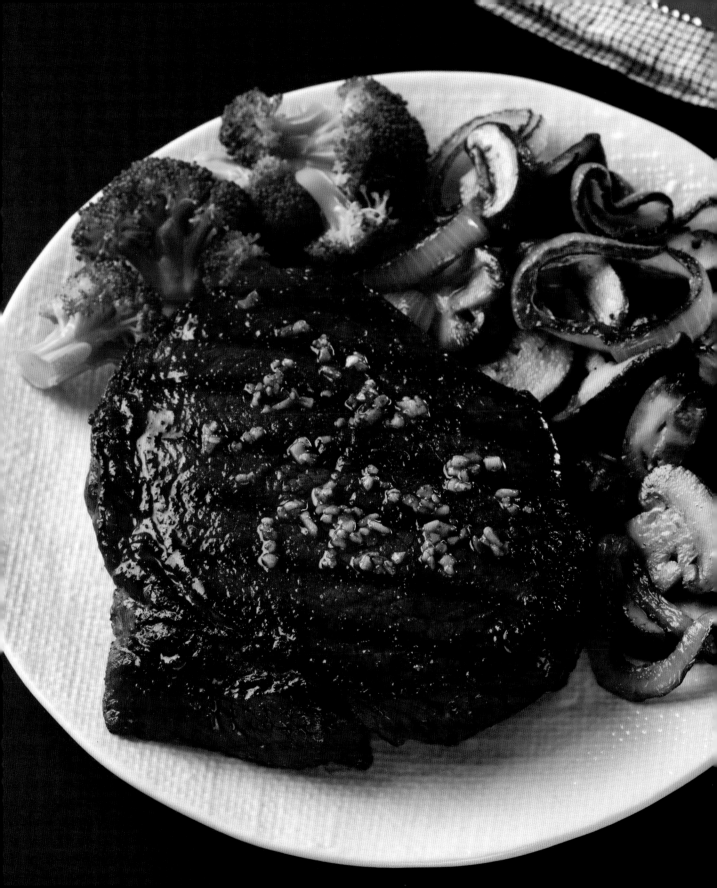

POULTRY

Sassy Chicken and Peppers

MAKES 4 SERVINGS

1 tablespoon Mexican seasoning*

4 boneless skinless chicken breasts (about 1 pound total)

1 tablespoon vegetable oil

1 red onion, sliced

1 medium red bell pepper, cut into thin strips

1 medium yellow or green bell pepper, cut into thin strips

½ cup chunky salsa or chipotle salsa

2 tablespoons lime juice

Lime wedges (optional)

Or substitute 1 teaspoon chili powder, ½ teaspoon ground cumin, ½ teaspoon salt and ⅛ teaspoon ground red pepper.

1 Sprinkle seasoning over both sides of chicken; set aside.

2 Heat oil in large nonstick skillet over medium heat. Add onion; cook 3 minutes, stirring occasionally.

3 Add bell peppers; cook 3 minutes, stirring occasionally. Stir salsa and lime juice into vegetables.

4 Push vegetables to edge of skillet. Add chicken to skillet. Cook 5 minutes; turn. Continue to cook 4 minutes or until chicken is no longer pink in center and vegetables are tender.

5 Serve chicken over vegetable mixture. Garnish with lime wedges.

NUTRIENTS PER SERVING

CALORIES 224

TOTAL FAT 8g

SATURATED FAT 1g

CHOLESTEROL 69mg

SODIUM 813mg

CARBOHYDRATE 11g

DIETARY FIBER 3g

PROTEIN 27g

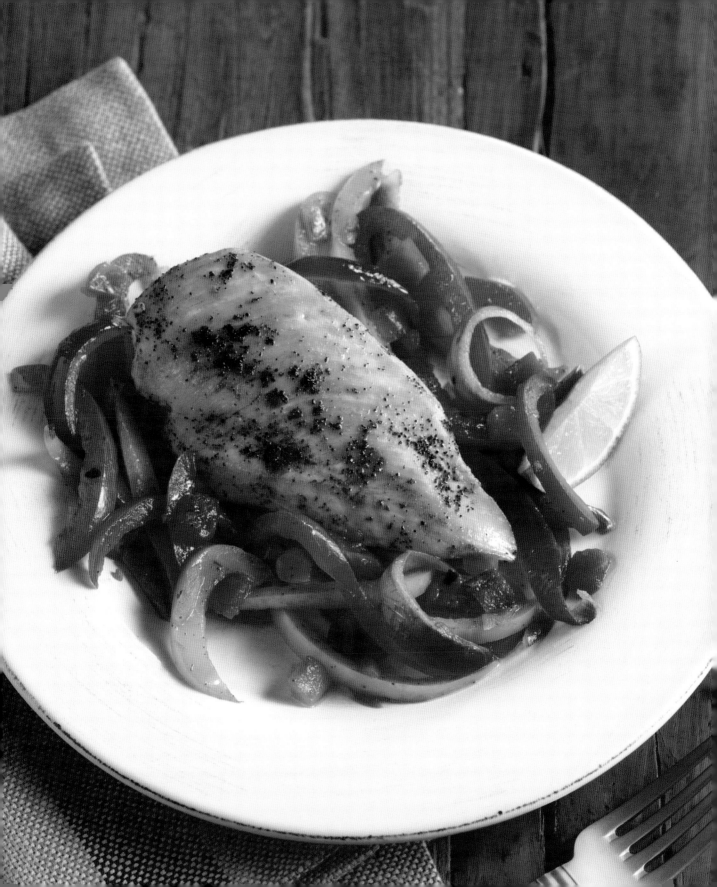

Quick and Easy Sautéed Chicken

MAKES 4 SERVINGS

NUTRIENTS
PER SERVING

CALORIES
147

TOTAL FAT
4g

SATURATED FAT
1g

CHOLESTEROL
66mg

SODIUM
242mg

CARBOHYDRATE
1g

DIETARY FIBER
1g

PROTEIN
26g

4   boneless skinless chicken breasts (4 ounces each)

1   teaspoon smoked or regular paprika

1   teaspoon dried thyme

½   teaspoon garlic salt

⅛   teaspoon ground red pepper

2   teaspoons olive oil

1 Place chicken breasts between sheets of waxed paper or plastic wrap; pound to even ½-inch thickness. Combine paprika, thyme, garlic salt and red pepper in small bowl; rub over both sides of chicken.

2 Heat oil in large nonstick skillet over medium heat. Add chicken; cook 4 to 5 minutes per side or until chicken is no longer pink in center. Pour any juices from skillet over chicken.

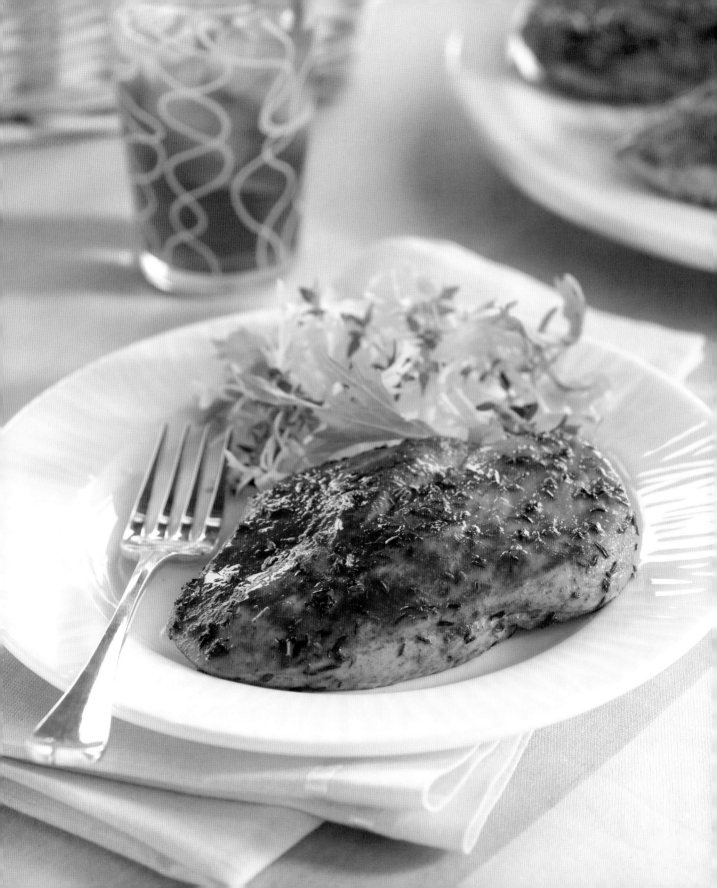

Prosciutto-Wrapped Chicken with Goat Cheese

MAKES 4 SERVINGS

8 slices lean prosciutto

4 boneless skinless chicken breasts (4 ounces each), pounded to ¼-inch thickness and cut in half crosswise

2 to 3 ounces goat cheese

24 basil leaves

1 teaspoon olive oil

1 shallot, finely chopped

2 tablespoons dry red wine

1 Preheat oven to 350°F. Coat 8-inch square baking pan with nonstick cooking spray.

2 Lay prosciutto on clean work surface or cutting board. Place chicken on top of each prosciutto piece. Top chicken with goat cheese. Place 3 basil leaves on top of each mound of cheese. Wrap prosciutto around chicken and secure with toothpicks in an X fashion. Place in prepared baking pan.

3 Heat oil in small skillet over medium heat. Add shallot; cook and stir about 2 minutes or until softened. Add wine; scrape up browned bits with wooden spoon. Pour shallot and wine over chicken. Bake 20 minutes or until chicken is cooked through.

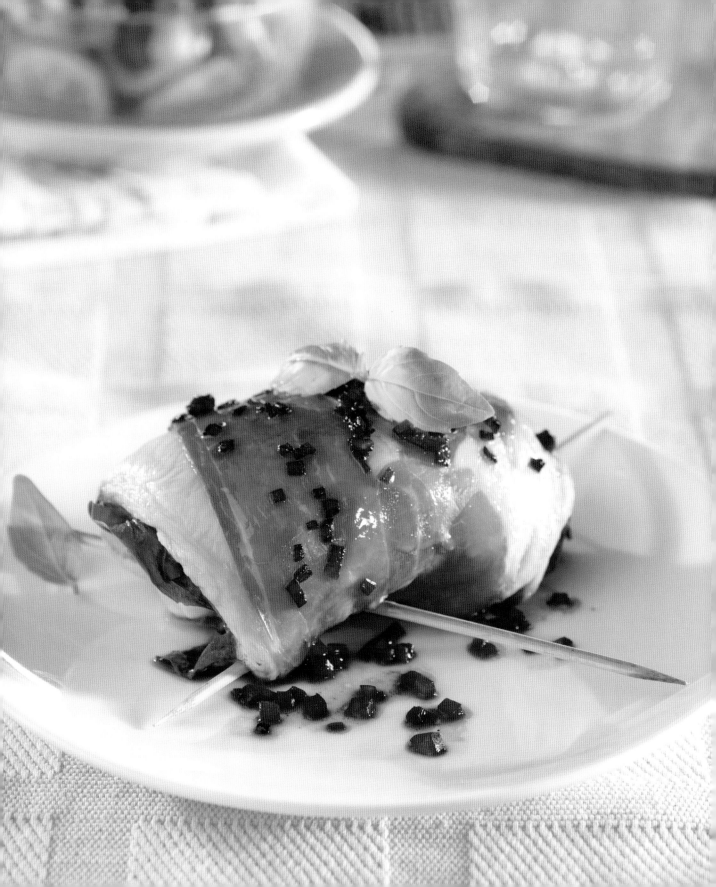

Southwest Chicken Burgers with Avocado Salad

NUTRIENTS PER SERVING

CALORIES
273

TOTAL FAT
11g

SATURATED FAT
3g

CHOLESTEROL
87mg

SODIUM
209mg

CARBOHYDRATE
9g

DIETARY FIBER
3g

PROTEIN
34g

MAKES 6 SERVINGS

1 cup finely diced yellow or red bell pepper, divided

½ cup finely diced red onion, divided

1 egg white

1½ teaspoons chili powder, divided

20 ounces ground chicken

1 medium avocado, diced

½ cup finely diced cucumber

Juice of 1 lime

4 tablespoons shredded Cheddar cheese

1 Combine ½ cup bell pepper, ¼ cup onion, egg white and 1 teaspoon chili powder in large bowl. Add chicken; stir to combine. Shape mixture into six patties. Cover and refrigerate 15 minutes.

2 Combine avocado, cucumber, lime juice, remaining ½ cup bell pepper, ¼ cup onion and ½ teaspoon chili powder in medium bowl.

3 Spray large skillet with nonstick cooking spray; heat over medium heat. Cook burgers 5 minutes. Turn and top each burger with cheese. Cook 5 minutes or until no longer pink in center.

4 Divide avocado salad among six plates; top with burgers.

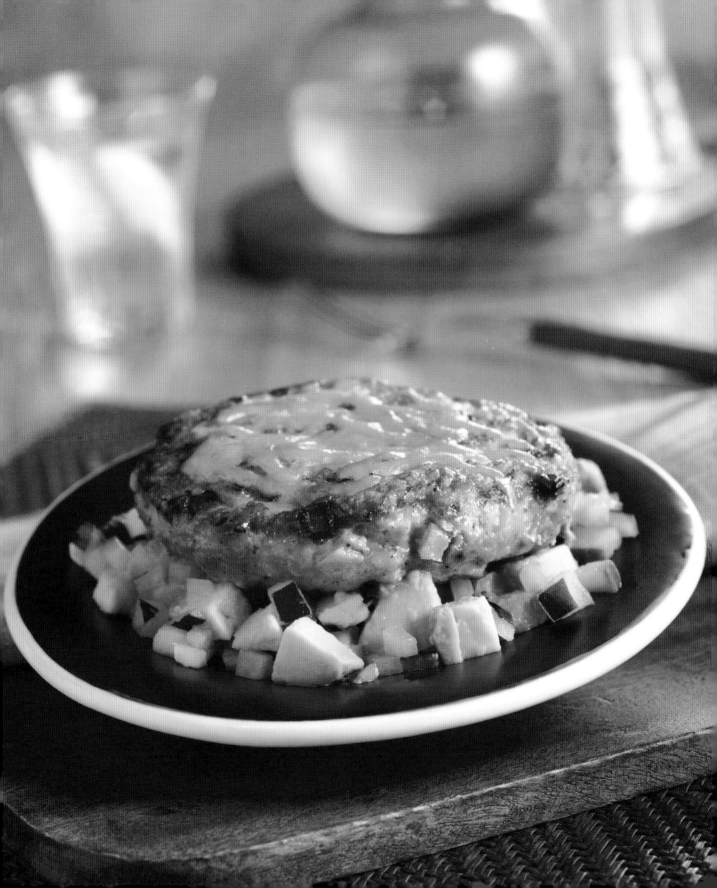

Grilled Chicken Adobo

MAKES 4 SERVINGS

NUTRIENTS
PER SERVING

CALORIES
139

TOTAL FAT
3g

SATURATED FAT
1g

CHOLESTEROL
69mg

SODIUM
61mg

CARBOHYDRATE
1g

DIETARY FIBER
1g

PROTEIN
25g

½ cup chopped onion

⅓ cup lime juice

6 cloves garlic, coarsely chopped

1 teaspoon ground cumin

1 teaspoon dried oregano

½ teaspoon dried thyme

¼ teaspoon ground red pepper

4 boneless skinless chicken breasts (about 1 pound total)

3 tablespoons chopped fresh cilantro (optional)

Salt and black pepper

1 Combine onion, lime juice and garlic in food processor. Process until onion is finely minced. Transfer to large resealable food storage bag. Add cumin, oregano, thyme and red pepper; knead bag until blended. Place chicken in bag; press out air and seal. Turn to coat chicken with marinade. Refrigerate 30 minutes or up to 4 hours, turning occasionally.

2 Spray grid with nonstick cooking spray. Prepare grill for direct cooking. Remove chicken from marinade; discard marinade. Place chicken on grid. Grill 5 to 7 minutes per side over medium heat or until chicken is no longer pink in center. Garnish with cilantro; season with salt and black pepper.

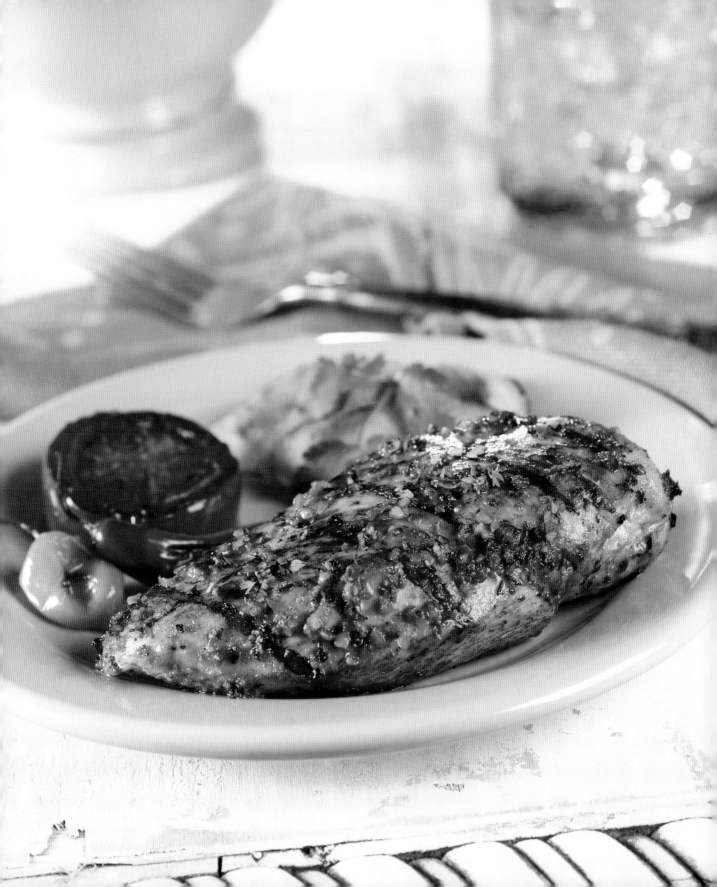

Spicy Lemony Almond Chicken

MAKES 4 SERVINGS

NUTRIENTS PER SERVING

CALORIES
193

TOTAL FAT
7g

SATURATED FAT
1g

CHOLESTEROL
66mg

SODIUM
257mg

CARBOHYDRATE
3g

DIETARY FIBER
1g

PROTEIN
28g

½ teaspoon paprika

½ teaspoon black pepper

¼ teaspoon salt

4 boneless skinless chicken breasts (about 1 pound total), flattened to ¼-inch thickness

Nonstick cooking spray *or* 2 teaspoons olive oil

1 ounce slivered almonds, toasted

¼ cup water

2 tablespoons lemon juice

2 tablespoons margarine or butter

2 teaspoons Worcestershire sauce

½ teaspoon grated lemon peel

1 Combine paprika, pepper and salt in small bowl; sprinkle evenly over both sides of chicken.

2 Coat large nonstick skillet with cooking spray or place oil in skillet; heat over medium-high heat. Add chicken; cook 3 to 4 minutes per side or until no longer pink in center. Set aside on serving platter. Sprinkle with almonds; cover to keep warm.

3 Add water, lemon juice, margarine and Worcestershire sauce to skillet. Cook until reduced to ¼ cup, scraping bottom and side of skillet. Remove from heat; stir in lemon peel. Spoon evenly over chicken.

TIP

To pound chicken, place between two pieces of plastic wrap. Starting in the center, pound chicken with a meat mallet to reach an even thickness.

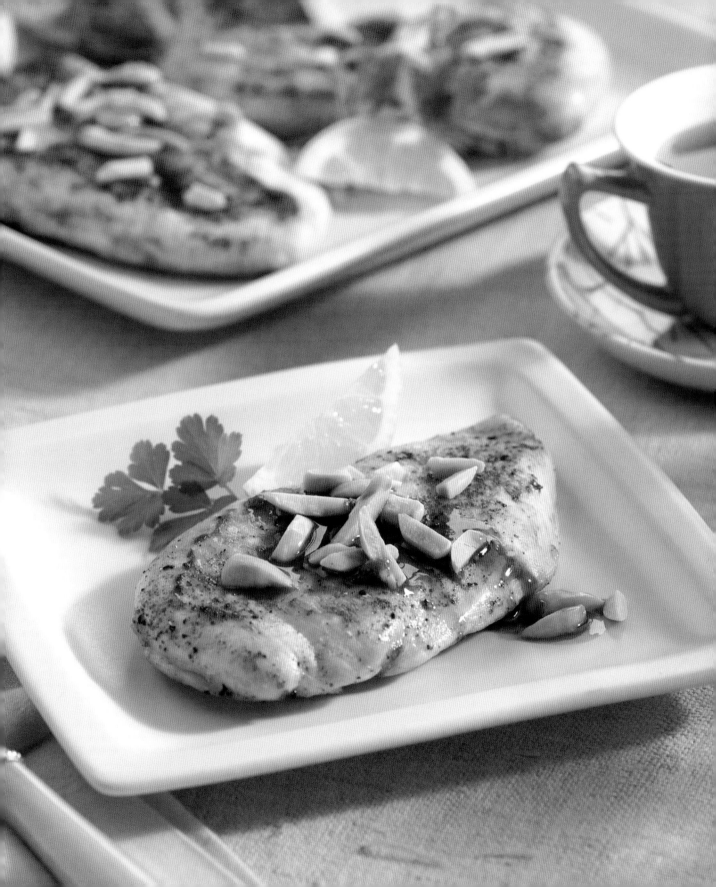

Greek Chicken Burgers with Cucumber Yogurt Sauce

MAKES 4 SERVINGS

½ cup plus 2 tablespoons plain nonfat or regular Greek yogurt

½ medium cucumber, peeled, seeded and finely chopped

Juice of ½ lemon

3 cloves garlic, minced, divided

2 teaspoons finely chopped fresh mint *or* ½ teaspoon dried mint

⅛ teaspoon salt

⅛ teaspoon ground white pepper

1 pound ground chicken breast

3 ounces reduced-fat or regular crumbled feta cheese

4 large kalamata olives, rinsed, patted dry and minced

1 egg

½ to 1 teaspoon dried oregano

¼ teaspoon black pepper

Mixed baby lettuce (optional)

1 Combine yogurt, cucumber, lemon juice, 2 cloves garlic, mint, salt and white pepper in medium bowl; mix well. Cover and refrigerate until ready to serve.

2 Combine chicken, cheese, olives, egg, oregano, black pepper and remaining 1 clove garlic in large bowl; mix well. Shape mixture into four patties.

3 Spray grill pan with nonstick cooking spray; heat over medium-high heat. Grill patties 5 to 7 minutes per side or until cooked through (165°F). Serve burgers with sauce and mixed greens, if desired.

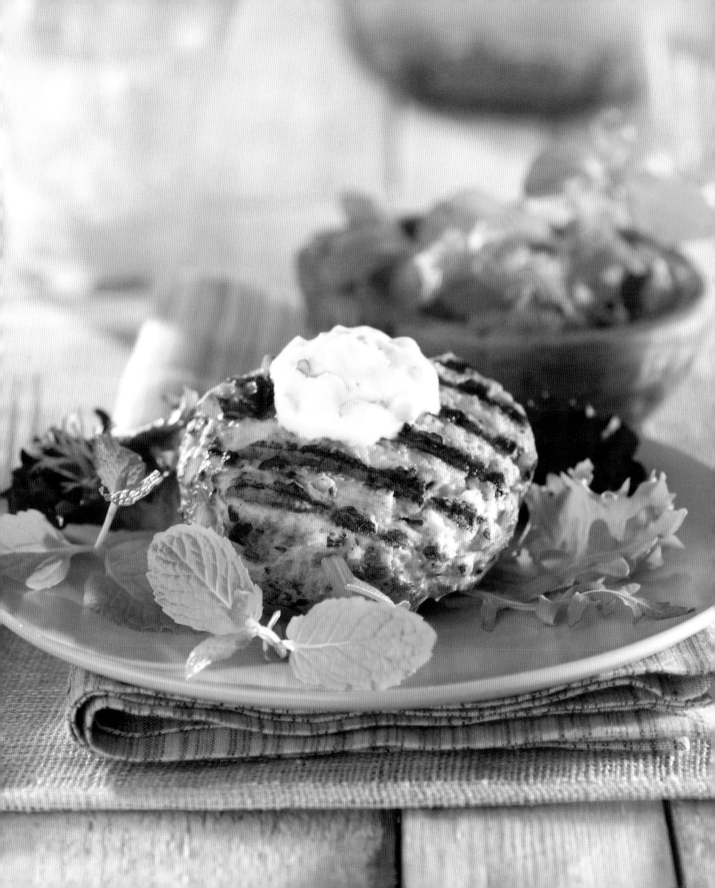

Chicken Scarpiello

MAKES 6 SERVINGS

3 tablespoons extra virgin olive oil, divided

1 pound spicy Italian sausage, cut into 1-inch pieces

1 cut-up whole chicken (about 3 pounds)*

1 teaspoon salt, divided

1 large onion, chopped

2 red, yellow or orange bell peppers, cut into ¼-inch strips

3 cloves garlic, minced

½ cup dry white wine

½ cup chicken broth

½ cup coarsely chopped seeded hot cherry peppers

½ cup liquid from cherry pepper jar

1 teaspoon dried oregano

Additional salt and black pepper

¼ cup chopped fresh Italian parsley

Or purchase 2 bone-in chicken leg quarters and 2 chicken breasts; separate drumsticks and thighs and cut breasts in half.

1 Heat 1 tablespoon oil in large skillet over medium-high heat. Add sausage; cook about 10 minutes or until well browned on all sides, stirring occasionally. Remove sausage from skillet; set aside.

2 Heat 1 tablespoon oil in same skillet. Sprinkle chicken with ½ teaspoon salt; arrange skin side down in single layer in skillet (cook in batches if necessary). Cook about 6 minutes per side or until browned. Remove chicken from skillet; set aside. Drain oil from skillet.

3 Heat remaining 1 tablespoon oil in skillet. Add onion and remaining ½ teaspoon salt; cook and stir 2 minutes or until onion is softened, scraping up browned bits from bottom of skillet. Add bell peppers and garlic; cook and stir 5 minutes. Stir in wine; cook until liquid is reduced by half. Stir in broth, cherry peppers, cherry pepper liquid, oregano and salt and black pepper to taste; bring to a simmer.

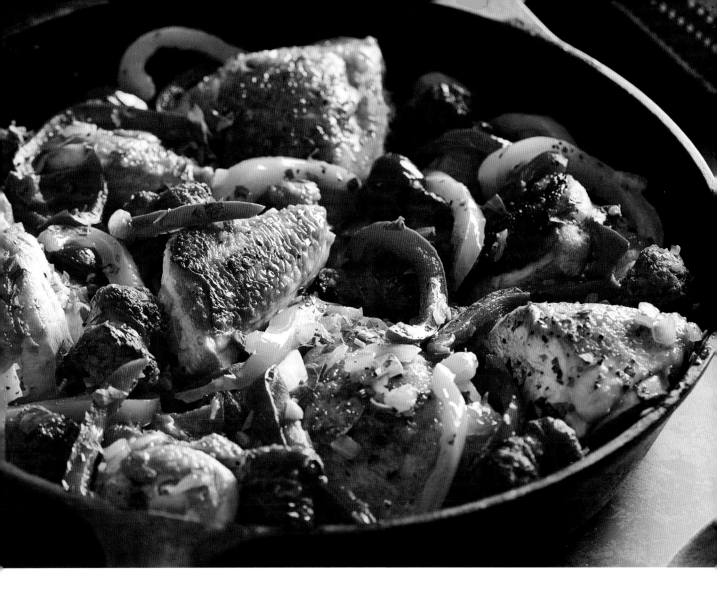

4 Return sausage and chicken along with any accumulated juices to skillet. Partially cover skillet and simmer 10 minutes. Uncover and simmer 15 minutes or until chicken is cooked through (165°F). Sprinkle with parsley.

TIP

If too much liquid remains in the skillet when the chicken is cooked through, remove the chicken and sausage and continue simmering the sauce to reduce it slightly.

Balsamic Chicken

MAKES 6 SERVINGS

1½ teaspoons fresh rosemary leaves, minced, *or* ½ teaspoon dried rosemary

2 cloves garlic, minced

¾ teaspoon black pepper

½ teaspoon salt

6 boneless skinless chicken breasts (about 1½ pounds total)

1 tablespoon olive oil

¼ cup balsamic vinegar

1 Combine rosemary, garlic, pepper and salt in small bowl; mix well. Place chicken in large bowl; drizzle with oil and rub with spice mixture. Cover and refrigerate 1 to 3 hours.

2 Preheat oven to 450°F. Spray 13×9-inch baking pan with nonstick cooking spray. Place chicken in pan; bake 10 minutes. Turn chicken over, stirring in 3 to 4 tablespoons water if drippings begin to stick to pan.

3 Bake about 10 minutes or until chicken is golden brown and no longer pink in center. If pan is dry, stir in another 1 to 2 tablespoons water.

4 Drizzle vinegar over chicken in pan. Remove chicken to plates. Stir liquid in pan; drizzle over chicken.

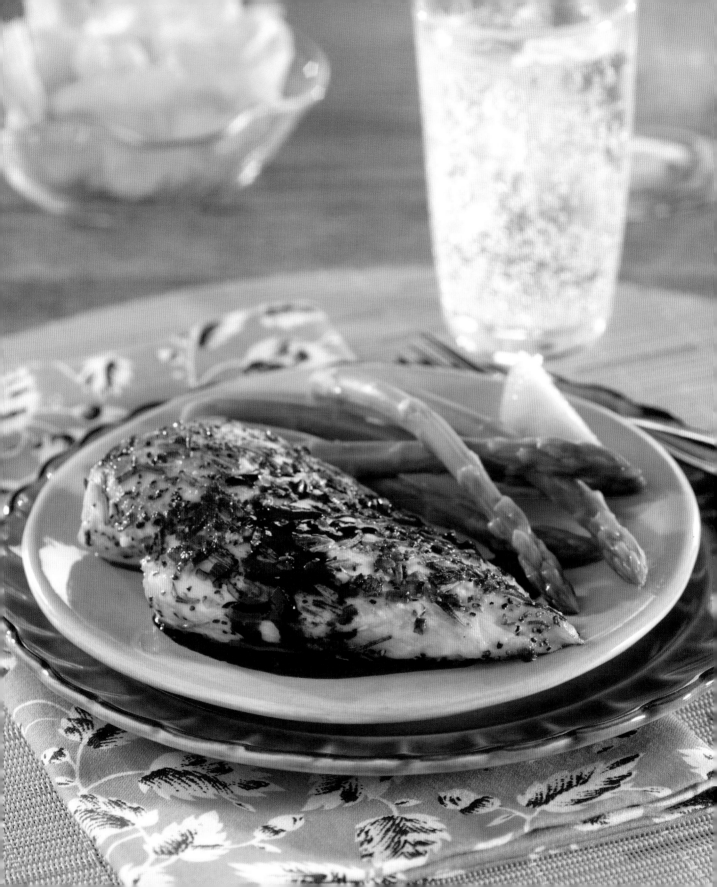

Jalapeño-Lime Chicken

MAKES 8 SERVINGS

NUTRIENTS PER SERVING

CALORIES
467

TOTAL FAT
32g

SATURATED FAT
9g

CHOLESTEROL
158mg

SODIUM
221mg

CARBOHYDRATE
11g

DIETARY FIBER
1g

PROTEIN
33g

8 chicken thighs

3 tablespoons jalapeño jelly

1 tablespoon olive oil

1 tablespoon lime juice

1 clove garlic, minced

1 teaspoon chili powder

½ teaspoon black pepper

⅛ teaspoon salt

1 Preheat oven to 400°F. Line 15×10-inch jelly-roll pan with foil; spray with nonstick cooking spray.

2 Arrange chicken in single layer in prepared pan. Bake 15 minutes; drain off juices.

3 Combine jelly, oil, lime juice, garlic, chili powder, pepper and salt in small bowl. Turn chicken; brush with half of jelly mixture. Bake 20 minutes. Turn chicken; brush with remaining jelly mixture. Bake chicken 10 to 15 minutes or until cooked through (180°F).

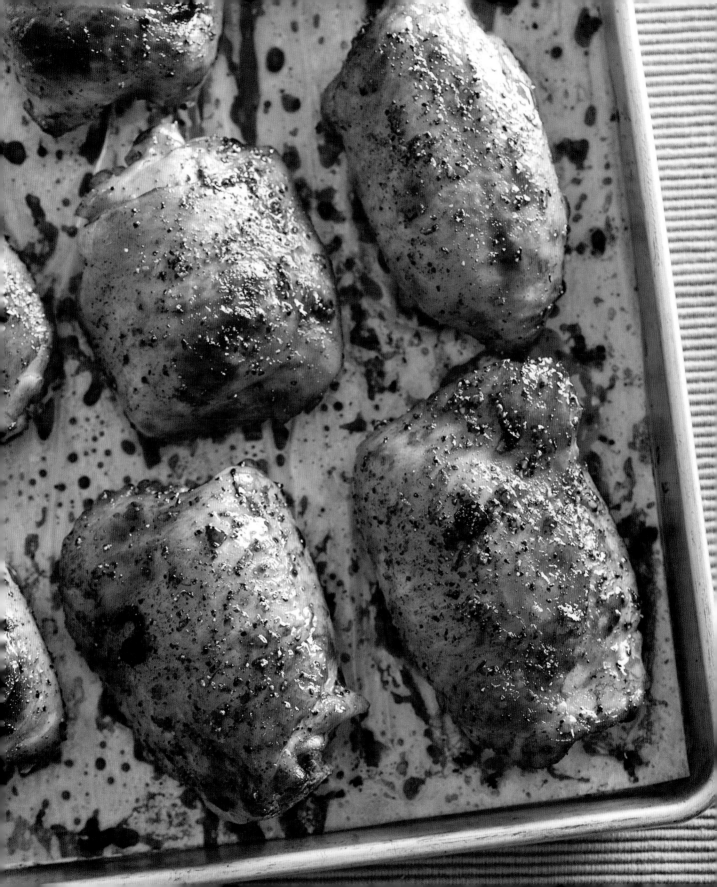

Chicken Piccata

MAKES 4 SERVINGS

3 tablespoons almond flour

½ teaspoon salt

¼ teaspoon black pepper

4 boneless skinless chicken breasts (about 1 pound total)

2 teaspoons olive oil

1 teaspoon butter

2 cloves garlic, minced

¾ cup reduced-sodium chicken broth

1 tablespoon fresh lemon juice

2 tablespoons chopped fresh Italian parsley

1 tablespoon capers, drained

1 Combine almond flour, salt and pepper in shallow dish. Reserve 1 tablespoon flour mixture.

2 Pound chicken between waxed paper to ½-inch thickness with flat side of meat mallet or rolling pin. Coat chicken with remaining flour mixture, shaking off excess.

3 Heat oil and butter in large nonstick skillet over medium heat. Add chicken; cook 4 to 5 minutes per side or until no longer pink in center. Transfer to serving platter; cover loosely with foil.

4 Add garlic to same skillet; cook and stir 1 minute. Add reserved flour mixture; cook and stir 1 minute. Add broth and lemon juice; cook 2 minutes or until thickened, stirring frequently. Stir in parsley and capers; spoon sauce over chicken.

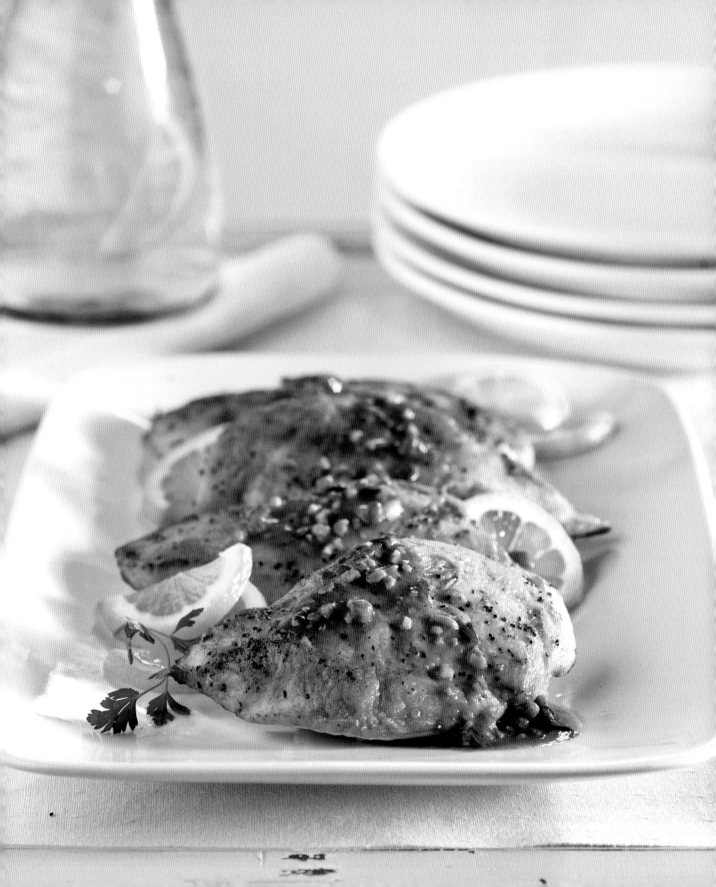

Blue Cheese Stuffed Chicken Breasts

MAKES 4 SERVINGS

½ cup (2 ounces) crumbled blue cheese

2 tablespoons butter, softened, divided

¾ teaspoon dried thyme

Salt and black pepper

4 bone-in skin-on chicken breasts

1 tablespoon lemon juice

½ teaspoon paprika

1 Prepare grill for direct cooking. Combine blue cheese, 1 tablespoon butter and thyme in small bowl until blended. Season with salt and pepper.

2 Loosen skin over chicken by pushing fingers between skin and meat, taking care not to tear skin. Spread blue cheese mixture under skin; massage skin to evenly spread cheese mixture.

3 Place chicken, skin side down, on grid over medium coals. Grill, covered, 15 minutes. Meanwhile, melt remaining 1 tablespoon butter; stir in lemon juice and paprika. Turn chicken; brush with butter mixture. Grill 15 to 20 minutes or until chicken is cooked through (165°F).

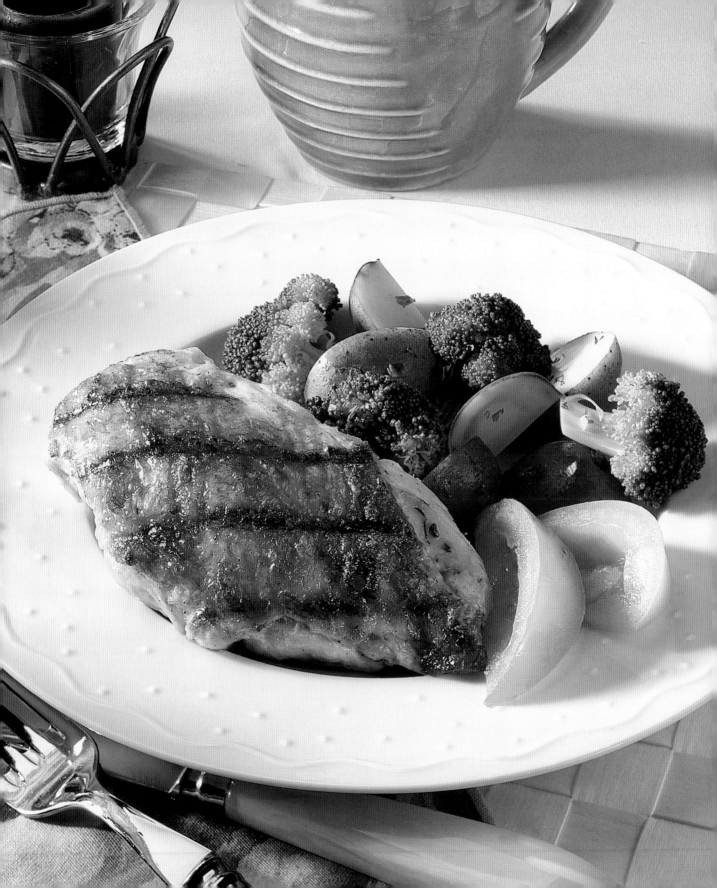

Crispy Roasted Chicken

MAKES 8 SERVINGS

1 roasting chicken or capon
  (about 6½ pounds)

1 tablespoon peanut or
  vegetable oil

2 cloves garlic, minced

1 tablespoon soy sauce

1 Preheat oven to 350°F. Place chicken on rack in shallow, foil-lined roasting pan.

2 Combine oil and garlic in small cup; brush evenly over chicken. Roast 15 to 20 minutes per pound or until internal temperature reaches 170°F when tested with meat thermometer inserted into thickest part of thigh not touching bone.

3 *Increase oven temperature to 450°F.* Remove drippings from pan; discard. Brush chicken evenly with soy sauce. Roast 5 to 10 minutes until skin is very crisp and deep golden brown. Transfer chicken to cutting board; let stand 10 to 15 minutes before carving. Internal temperature will continue to rise 5° to 10°F during stand time. Cover and refrigerate leftovers up to 3 days or freeze up to 3 months.

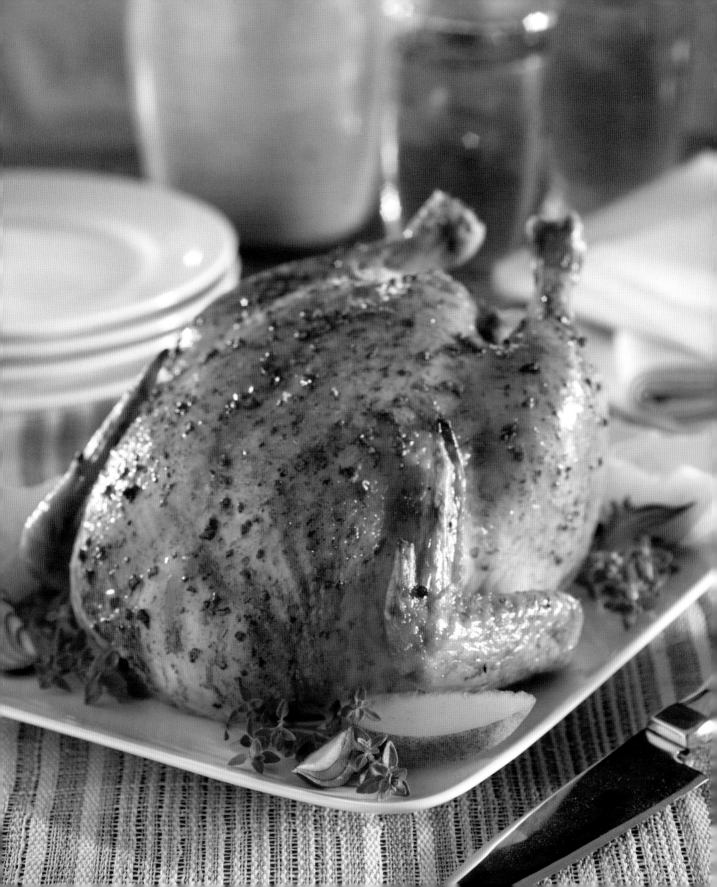

Cilantro-Stuffed Chicken Breasts

MAKES 4 SERVINGS

2 cloves garlic

1 cup packed fresh cilantro leaves

1 tablespoon plus 2 teaspoons soy sauce, divided

1 tablespoon peanut or vegetable oil

4 boneless skin-on chicken breasts (about 1¼ pounds total)

1 tablespoon dark sesame oil

1 Preheat oven to 350°F. Place garlic in food processor; process until minced. Add cilantro; process until cilantro is minced. Add 2 teaspoons soy sauce and peanut oil; process until paste forms.

2 With rubber spatula or fingers, distribute about 1 tablespoon cilantro mixture evenly under skin of each chicken breast half, taking care not to puncture skin.

3 Place chicken on rack in shallow, foil-lined baking pan. Combine remaining 1 tablespoon soy sauce and sesame oil. Brush half of mixture evenly over chicken. Bake 25 minutes; brush remaining soy sauce mixture evenly over chicken. Bake 10 minutes or until juices run clear.

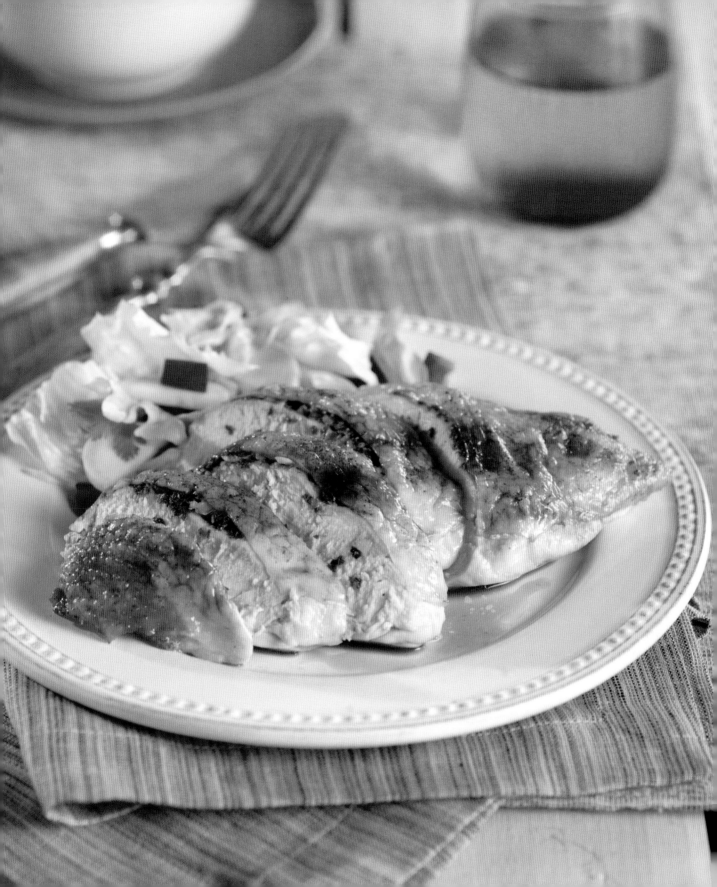

Forty-Clove Chicken Filice

MAKES 6 SERVINGS

¼ cup olive oil

1 whole chicken (about 3 pounds), cut into serving pieces

40 cloves garlic (about 2 heads), peeled

4 stalks celery, thickly sliced

½ cup dry white wine

¼ cup dry vermouth

Grated peel and juice of 1 lemon

2 tablespoons finely chopped fresh parsley

2 teaspoons dried basil

1 teaspoon dried oregano, crushed

Pinch of red pepper flakes

Salt and black pepper

1 Preheat oven to 375°F.

2 Heat oil in Dutch oven. Add chicken; cook until browned on all sides.

3 Combine garlic, celery, wine, vermouth, lemon juice, parsley, basil, oregano and red pepper flakes in medium bowl; pour over chicken. Sprinkle with lemon peel; season with salt and black pepper.

4 Cover and bake 40 minutes. Remove cover; bake 15 minutes or until chicken is cooked through (165°F).

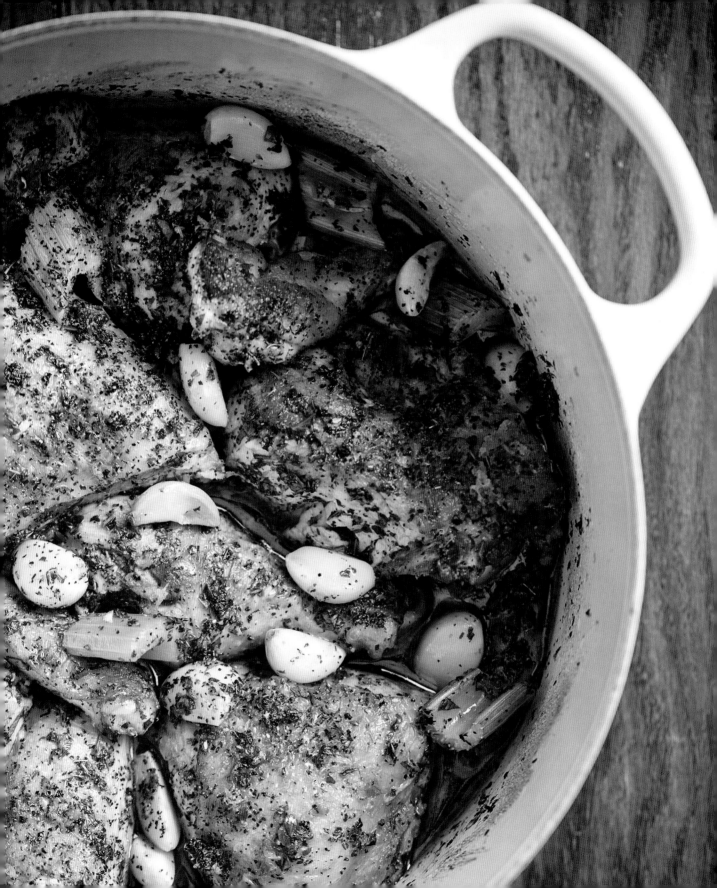

Lemony Greek Chicken

MAKES 4 SERVINGS

1 whole chicken (about 3 to 4 pounds), into serving pieces

1 tablespoon olive oil

2 teaspoons Greek seasoning

1 teaspoon salt

1 teaspoon black pepper

Juice of 1 lemon

1 Preheat oven to 400°F.

2 Brush chicken with oil. Arrange in two large baking dishes, bone side down. Combine Greek seasoning, salt and pepper in small bowl; sprinkle half over chicken. Bake 30 minutes.

3 Turn chicken pieces over. Sprinkle with remaining seasoning mixture and lemon juice. Bake 30 minutes or until chicken is cooked through (165°F).

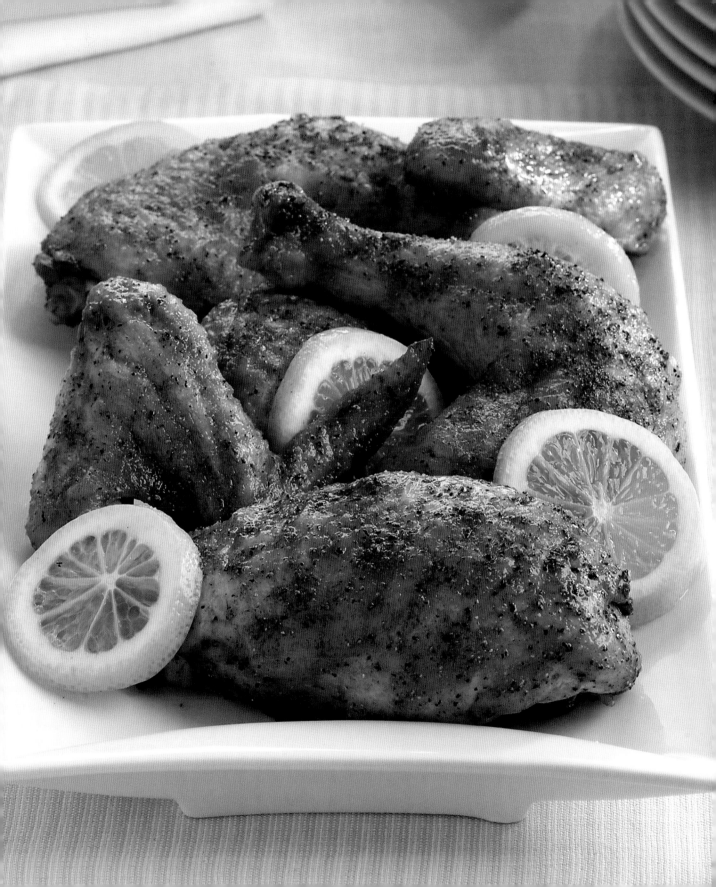

Kale and Mushroom Stuffed Chicken Breasts

MAKES 4 SERVINGS

NUTRIENTS PER SERVING

CALORIES
192

TOTAL FAT
7g

SATURATED FAT
1g

CHOLESTEROL
73mg

SODIUM
495mg

CARBOHYDRATE
4g

DIETARY FIBER
1g

PROTEIN
29g

3 teaspoons olive oil, divided

1 cup coarsely chopped mushrooms

2 cups thinly sliced kale

1 tablespoon fresh lemon juice

½ teaspoon salt, divided

4 boneless skinless chicken breasts (about 1 pound total)

¼ cup crumbled fat-free or regular feta cheese

¼ teaspoon black pepper

1 Heat 1 teaspoon oil in large skillet over medium-high heat. Add mushrooms; cook and stir 5 minutes or until mushrooms begin to brown. Add kale; cook and stir 8 minutes or until wilted. Sprinkle with lemon juice and ¼ teaspoon salt. Remove to small bowl. Let stand 5 to 10 minutes to cool slightly.

2 Meanwhile, place each chicken breast between sheets of plastic wrap. Pound with meat mallet or rolling pin to about ½-inch thickness.

3 Gently stir feta cheese into mushroom and kale mixture. Spoon ¼ cup mixture down center of each chicken breast. Roll up to enclose filling; secure with toothpicks. Sprinkle with remaining ¼ teaspoon salt and pepper.

4 Wipe out same skillet with paper towels. Add remaining 2 teaspoons oil to skillet; heat over medium heat. Add chicken; brown on all sides. Cover and cook 5 minutes per side or until no longer pink. Remove toothpicks before serving.

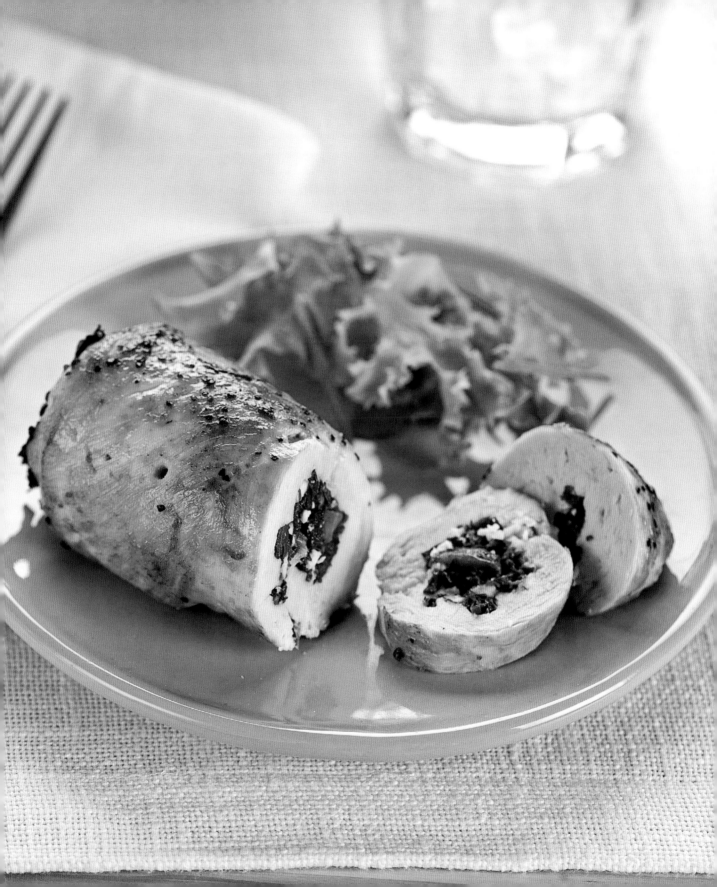

Creamy Baked Chicken with Artichokes and Mushrooms

MAKES 6 SERVINGS

6 boneless skinless chicken breasts (about 4 ounces each)

1½ teaspoons paprika

1½ teaspoons dried thyme

½ teaspoon salt

½ teaspoon black pepper

1 can (14 ounces) artichokes packed in water, drained

1 tablespoon butter

1 package (8 ounces) sliced cremini mushrooms

2 tablespoons almond meal

¾ cup reduced-sodium chicken broth

½ cup half-and-half

1 Preheat oven to 375°F.

2 Place chicken in 13×9-inch baking dish. Combine paprika, thyme, salt and pepper in small bowl; mix well. Reserve 1 teaspoon seasoning mixture; set aside. Sprinkle remaining seasoning mixture evenly over chicken. Cut artichokes in half; arrange around chicken.

3 Melt butter in large saucepan over medium heat. Add mushrooms and reserved 1 teaspoon seasoning mixture; cook and stir 5 minutes or until tender. Sprinkle almond meal over mushrooms; cook and stir 1 minute. Stir in broth; simmer 3 minutes or until thickened. Stir in half-and-half; cook 1 minute. Pour evenly over chicken and artichokes.

4 Bake 30 minutes or until chicken is no longer pink.

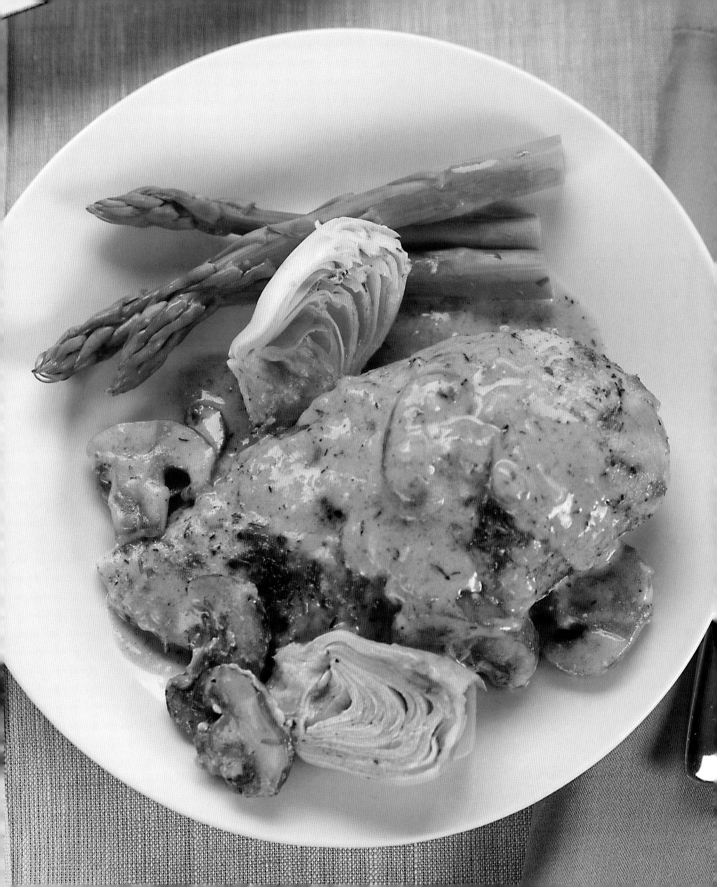

NUTRIENTS PER SERVING

CALORIES	230
TOTAL FAT	6g
SATURATED FAT	1g
CHOLESTEROL	95mg
SODIUM	400mg
CARBOHYDRATE	7g
DIETARY FIBER	2g
PROTEIN	36g

Chili Roasted Turkey with Cilantro-Lime Butternut Squash

MAKES 12 SERVINGS

TURKEY

- 1½ tablespoons chili powder
- 2 teaspoons dried oregano
- 1½ teaspoons ground cumin
- ½ teaspoon red pepper flakes
- ½ teaspoon salt
- ½ teaspoon black pepper
- 1 bone-in turkey breast with skin (5 pounds)

SQUASH

- 1 butternut squash, peeled and seeded
- 2 medium red bell peppers, julienned
- 2½ cups water
- ½ teaspoon ground turmeric
- 1 cup chopped green onions
- ½ cup chopped fresh cilantro
- 3 tablespoons olive oil
- 2 to 3 tablespoons lime juice
- 1 tablespoon grated lime peel
- ¾ teaspoon salt

1 Preheat oven to 325°F. Spray roasting pan and rack with nonstick cooking spray. Combine chili powder, oregano, cumin, pepper flakes, salt and black pepper in small bowl.

2 Separate turkey skin from meat by sliding fingers under skin. Spread chili mixture evenly over meat; cover with skin. (If skin tears, use toothpick to hold skin together.) Place turkey breast on prepared rack in roasting pan, skin side up.

3 Roast 1 hour and 30 minutes or until meat thermometer reaches 165°F. Remove from oven. Cover loosely with foil; let stand 10 to 15 minutes. Remove and discard skin, if desired.

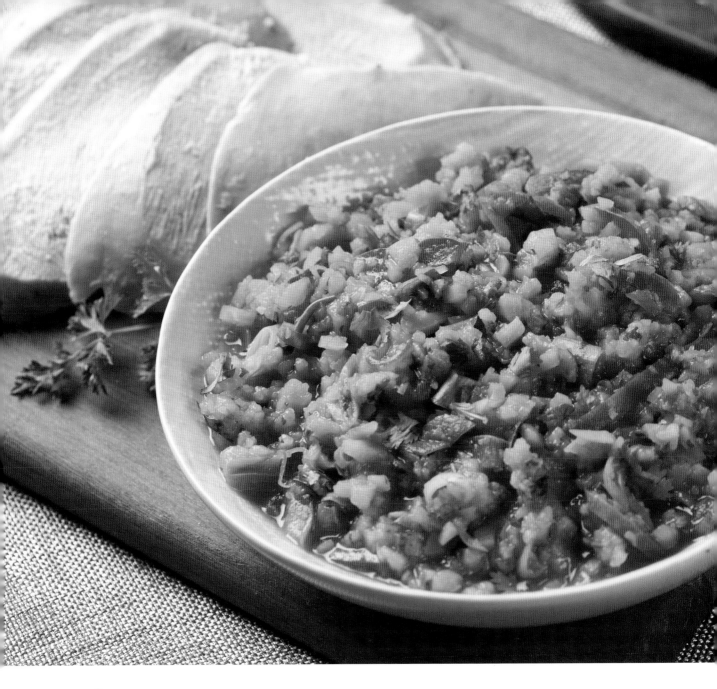

4 Meanwhile, cut squash into 1-inch pieces; place in food processor. Pulse until small pieces form. Combine bell peppers, water, squash and turmeric in large saucepan. Bring to a boil. Reduce heat; cover and simmer 10 minutes or until liquid has evaporated. Remove from heat; stir in green onions, cilantro, oil, lime juice, lime peel and salt. Serve with turkey.

FISH AND SEAFOOD

Tilapia with Spinach and Feta

MAKES 2 SERVINGS

1 teaspoon olive oil

1 clove garlic, minced

4 cups baby spinach

2 skinless tilapia fillets or other mild white fish (4 ounces each)

¼ teaspoon black pepper

2 ounces reduced-fat or regular feta cheese, cut into 2 (3-inch) pieces

1 Preheat oven to 350°F. Spray baking sheet with nonstick cooking spray.

2 Heat oil in medium skillet over medium-low heat. Add garlic; cook and stir 30 seconds. Add spinach; cook just until wilted, stirring occasionally.

3 Arrange tilapia on prepared baking sheet; sprinkle with pepper. Place one piece of cheese on each fillet; top with spinach mixture. Fold one end of each fillet up and over filling; secure with toothpick. Repeat with opposite end of each fillet.

4 Bake 20 minutes or until fish begins to flake when tested with fork.

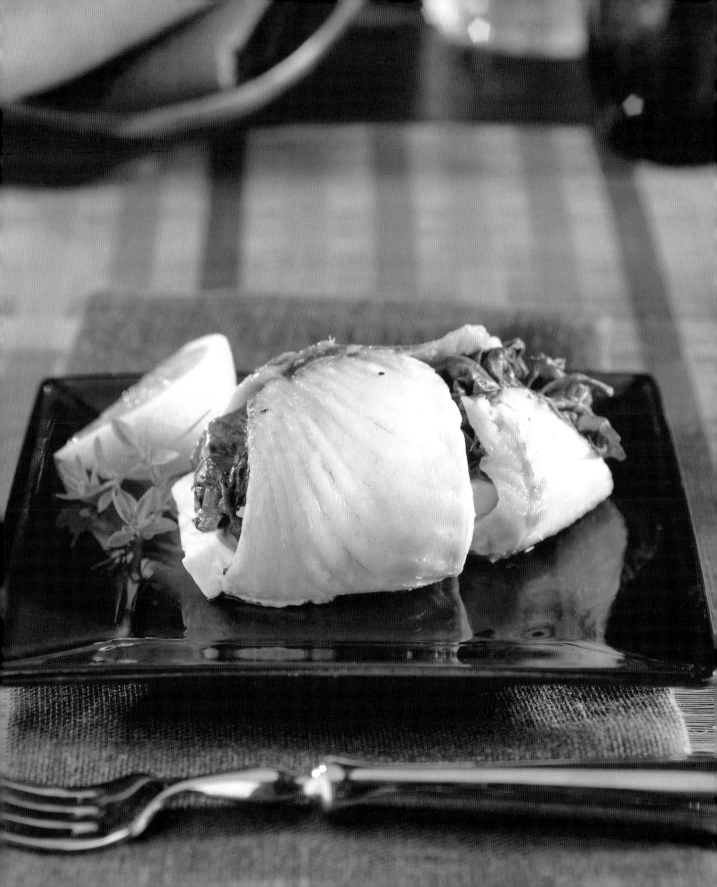

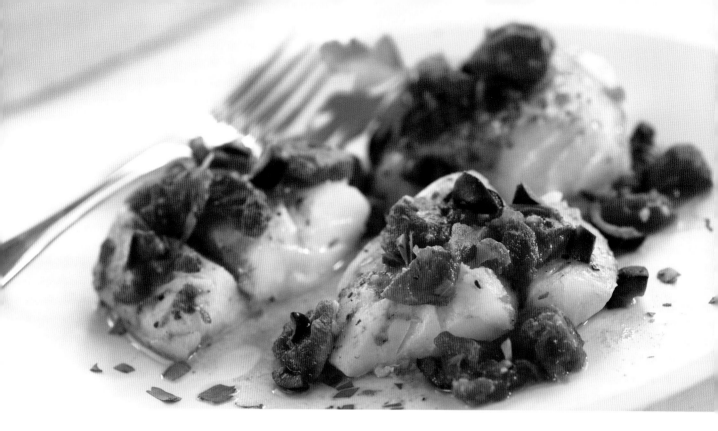

Baked Cod with Tomatoes and Olives

NUTRIENTS
PER SERVING

CALORIES
121

TOTAL FAT
1g

SATURATED FAT
1g

CHOLESTEROL
48mg

SODIUM
574mg

CARBOHYDRATE
5g

DIETARY FIBER
1g

PROTEIN
21g

MAKES 4 SERVINGS

4 cod fillets (about 4 ounces each), cut into 2-inch pieces

   Salt and black pepper

1 can (about 14 ounces) diced Italian-style tomatoes

2 tablespoons chopped pitted black olives

1 teaspoon minced garlic

2 tablespoons chopped fresh parsley

1 Preheat oven to 400°F. Spray 13×9-inch baking dish with nonstick olive oil-flavored cooking spray. Arrange cod fillets in dish; season with salt and pepper.

2 Combine tomatoes, olives and garlic in medium bowl. Spoon over fish.

3 Bake 20 minutes or until fish begins to flake when tested with fork. Sprinkle with parsley.

Dilled Salmon in Parchment

MAKES 2 SERVINGS

NUTRIENTS
PER SERVING

CALORIES
315

TOTAL FAT
24g

SATURATED FAT
10g

CHOLESTEROL
88mg

SODIUM
141mg

CARBOHYDRATE
2g

DIETARY FIBER
1g

PROTEIN
23g

2 skinless salmon fillets (4 to 6 ounces each)

2 tablespoons butter, melted

1 tablespoon lemon juice

1 tablespoon chopped fresh dill

1 tablespoon chopped shallots

Salt and black pepper

1 Preheat oven to 400°F. Cut two pieces of parchment paper into 12-inch squares; fold squares in half diagonally and cut into half heart shapes. Open parchment; place fish fillet on one side of each heart.

2 Combine butter and lemon juice in small bowl; drizzle over fish. Sprinkle with dill and shallots; season with salt and pepper.

3 Fold parchment hearts in half. Beginning at top of heart, fold edges together, 2 inches at a time. At tip of heart, fold parchment over to seal.

4 Bake fish about 10 minutes or until parchment pouch puffs up. To serve, cut an "X" through top layer of parchment and fold back points.

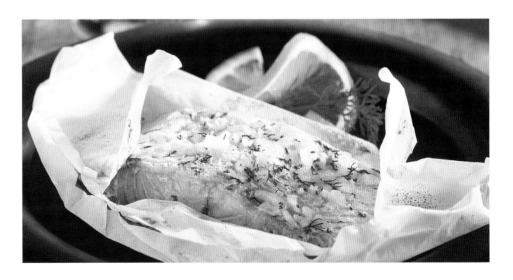

Blackened Shrimp with Tomatoes

MAKES 4 SERVINGS

NUTRIENTS PER SERVING

CALORIES
112

TOTAL FAT
5g

SATURATED FAT
1g

CHOLESTEROL
86mg

SODIUM
88mg

CARBOHYDRATE
5g

DIETARY FIBER
1g

PROTEIN
13g

1½ teaspoons paprika

1 teaspoon Italian seasoning

½ teaspoon garlic powder

¼ teaspoon black pepper

½ pound (about 24) small raw shrimp, peeled (with tails on)

1 tablespoon canola oil

1½ cups halved grape tomatoes

½ cup sliced onion, separated into rings

Lime wedges (optional)

1 Combine paprika, Italian seasoning, garlic powder and pepper in small bowl; place in large resealable food storage bag. Add shrimp; seal bag and shake to coat.

2 Heat oil in large skillet over medium-high heat. Add shrimp; cook 4 minutes or until shrimp are pink and opaque, turning occasionally.

3 Add tomatoes and onion to skillet; cook 1 minute or until tomatoes are heated through and onion is softened. Serve with lime wedges, if desired.

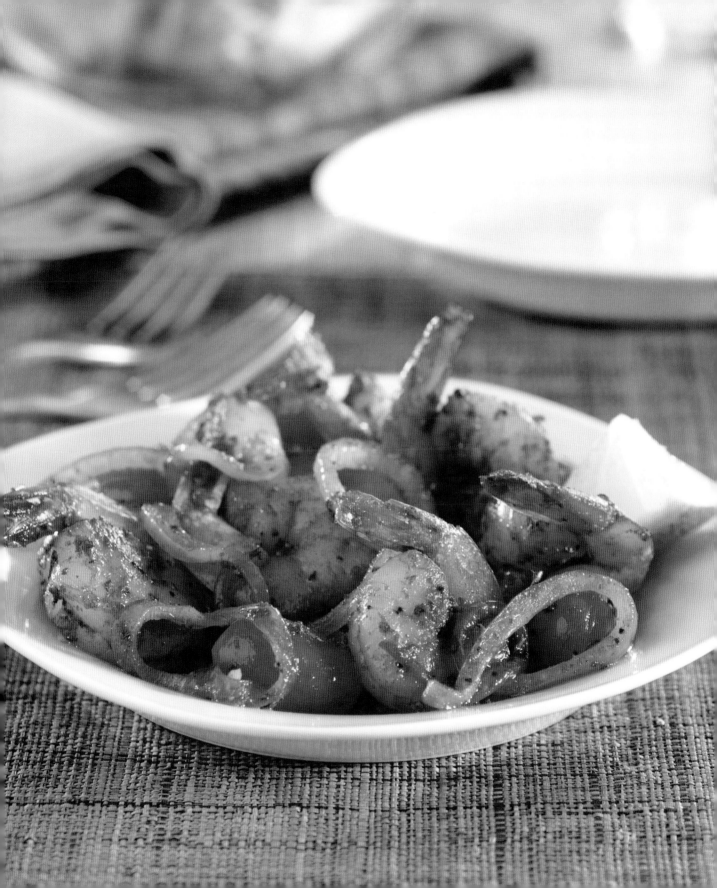

Seared Scallops Over Garlic-Lemon Spinach

MAKES 4 SERVINGS (ABOUT 3 SCALLOPS AND ¼ CUP SPINACH PER SERVING)

NUTRIENTS PER SERVING	
CALORIES	172
TOTAL FAT	5g
SATURATED FAT	1g
CHOLESTEROL	60mg
SODIUM	480mg
CARBOHYDRATE	3g
DIETARY FIBER	1g
PROTEIN	28g

1 tablespoon olive oil

1 pound sea scallops*
(approximately 12)

¼ teaspoon salt

⅛ teaspoon black pepper

2 cloves garlic, minced

1 shallot, minced

1 package (6 ounces) baby spinach

1 tablespoon fresh lemon juice

Lemon wedges (optional)

Make sure scallops are dry before putting them in the pan so they can get a golden crust.

1 Heat oil in large nonstick skillet over medium-high heat. Add scallops; sprinkle with salt and pepper. Cook 2 to 3 minutes per side or until golden. Remove to large plate; keep warm.

2 Add garlic and shallot to skillet; cook and stir 45 seconds or until fragrant. Add spinach; cook 2 minutes or until spinach just begins to wilt, stirring occasionally. Remove from heat; stir in lemon juice.

3 Serve scallops over spinach. Garnish with lemon wedges.

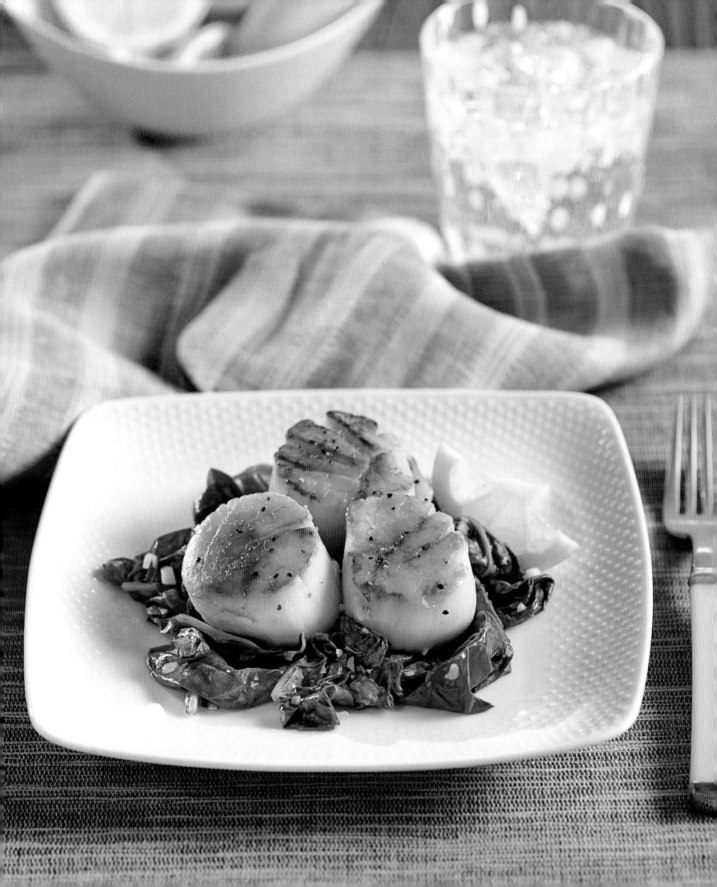

Salmon with Bok Choy

MAKES 4 SERVINGS

NUTRIENTS
PER SERVING

CALORIES
280

TOTAL FAT
15g

SATURATED FAT
3g

CHOLESTEROL
60mg

SODIUM
470mg

CARBOHYDRATE
9g

DIETARY FIBER
1g

PROTEIN
25g

4 skinless salmon fillets (about 4 ounces each)

3 tablespoons finely chopped fresh ginger

2 cloves garlic, minced

½ cup reduced-sodium vegetable broth

3 tablespoons unseasoned rice vinegar

1 tablespoon reduced-sodium soy sauce

6 cups chopped bok choy

1 teaspoon hoisin sauce

¼ cup sliced green onions

SLOW COOKER DIRECTIONS

1 Spray slow cooker with nonstick cooking spray. Arrange salmon in slow cooker; spread ginger and garlic evenly over salmon. Pour broth, vinegar and soy sauce over salmon. Cover; cook on LOW 1½ hours.

2 Add bok choy to slow cooker; cover and cook 30 minutes or until crisp-tender and salmon flakes easily when tested with fork.

3 Remove salmon from slow cooker; arrange on 4 plates. Stir hoisin sauce into liquid in slow cooker.

4 Spoon sauce evenly over salmon. Top with green onions. Serve with bok choy.

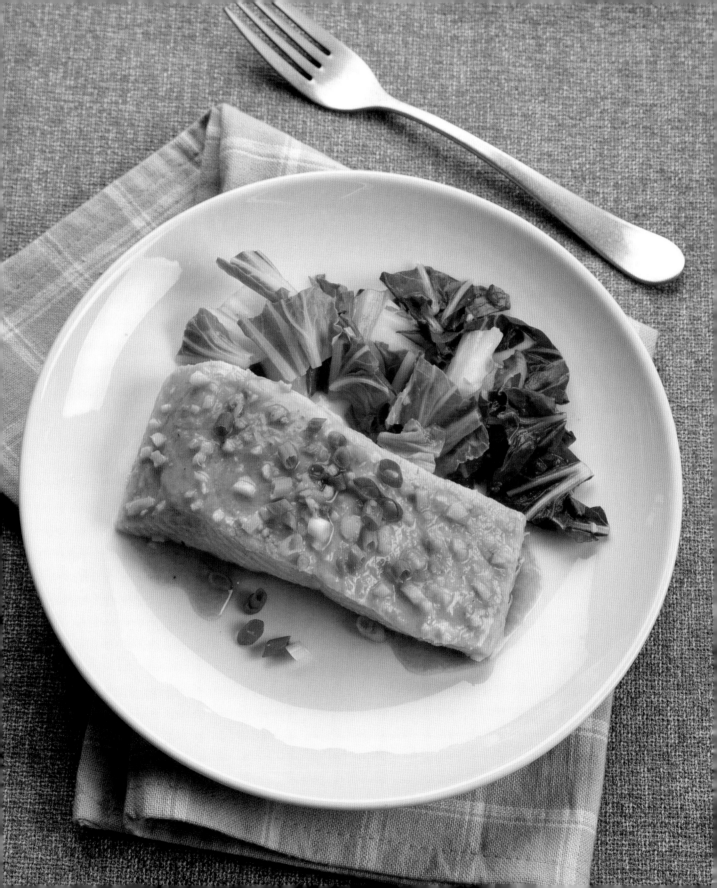

Roast Dill Scrod with Asparagus

MAKES 4 SERVINGS

NUTRIENTS PER SERVING	
CALORIES	147
TOTAL FAT	2g
SATURATED FAT	1g
CHOLESTEROL	61mg
SODIUM	379mg
CARBOHYDRATE	4g
DIETARY FIBER	2g
PROTEIN	27g

1 bunch (12 ounces) asparagus spears, ends trimmed
1 teaspoon olive oil
4 scrod or cod fillets (about 5 ounces each)
1 tablespoon lemon juice
1 teaspoon dried dill weed
½ teaspoon salt
¼ teaspoon black pepper
   Paprika (optional)

1 Preheat oven to 425°F.

2 Place asparagus in 13×9-inch baking dish; drizzle with oil. Roll asparagus to coat lightly with oil; push to edges of dish, stacking asparagus into two layers.

3 Arrange fish fillets in center of dish; drizzle with lemon juice. Combine dill, salt and pepper in small bowl; sprinkle over fish and asparagus. Sprinkle with paprika, if desired.

4 Roast 15 to 17 minutes or until asparagus is crisp-tender and fish is opaque in center and begins to flake when tested with fork.

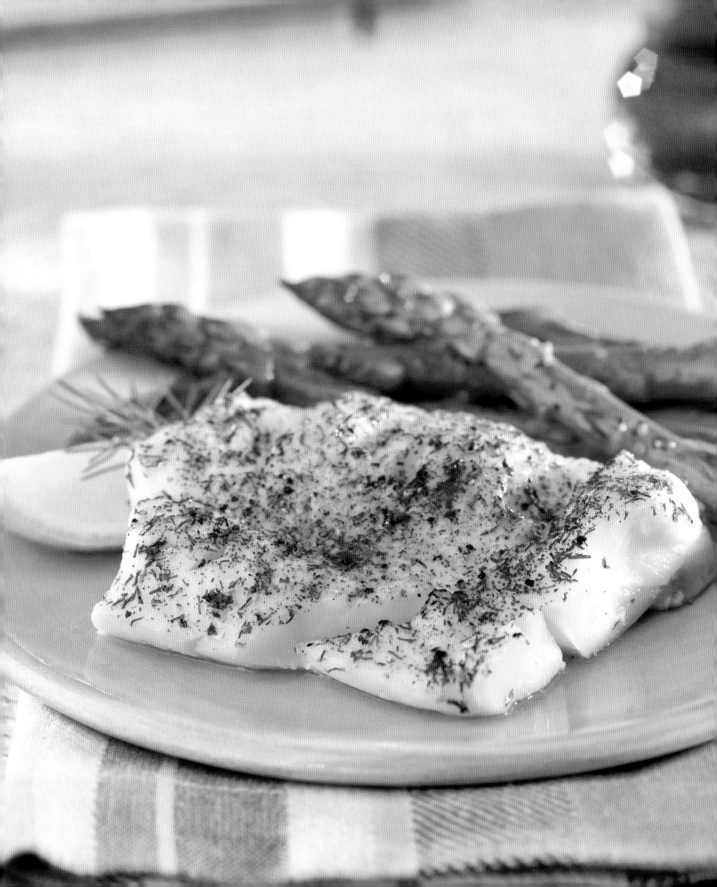

Trout Stuffed with Fresh Mint and Orange

MAKES 6 SERVINGS

2 pan-dressed* trout (1 to 1¼ pounds each)

½ teaspoon coarse salt

1 orange, sliced

1 cup fresh mint leaves

1 sweet onion, sliced

A pan-dressed trout has been gutted and scaled with head and tail removed.

1 Prepare grill for direct cooking.

2 Rinse trout under cold running water; pat dry with paper towels. Sprinkle cavities of trout with salt; fill each with orange slices and mint. Cover each fish with onion slices.

3 Spray two large sheets of foil with nonstick cooking spray. Place one fish on each sheet and seal using drugstore wrap technique.**

4 Place foil packets, seam side down, directly on medium-hot coals. Grill, covered, 20 to 25 minutes or until trout flakes easily when tested with fork, turning once.

5 Carefully open foil packets, avoiding hot steam; remove and discard orange-mint stuffing. Serve immediately.

**See tip on page 234.

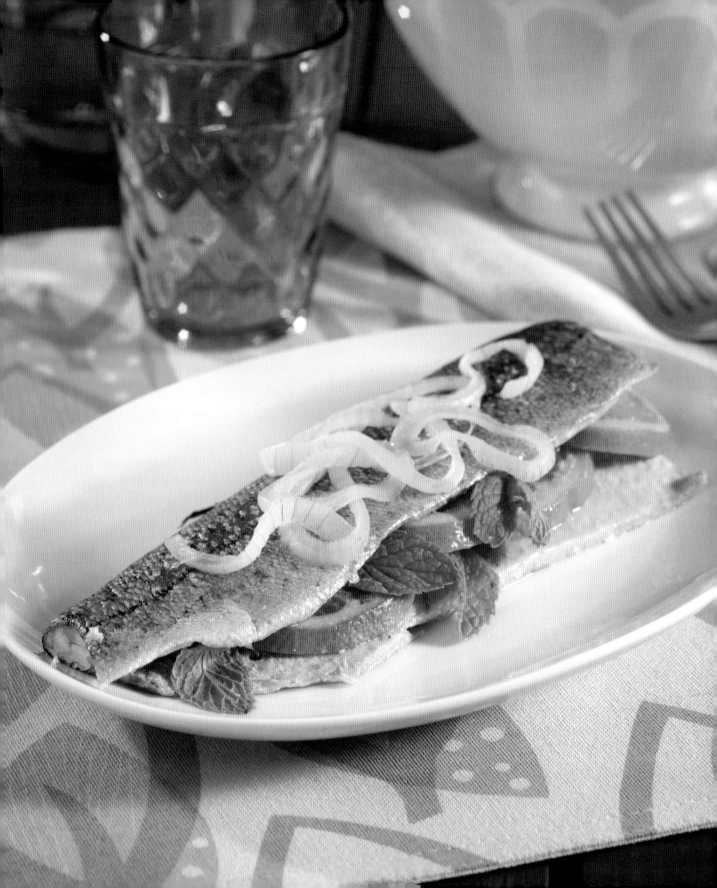

Grilled Five-Spice Fish with Garlic Spinach

MAKES 4 SERVINGS

NUTRIENTS
PER SERVING

CALORIES
241

TOTAL FAT
15g

SATURATED FAT
3g

CHOLESTEROL
66mg

SODIUM
426mg

CARBOHYDRATE
3g

DIETARY FIBER
1g

PROTEIN
24g

1½ teaspoons grated lime peel

3 tablespoons fresh lime juice

4 teaspoons minced fresh ginger

½ to 1 teaspoon Chinese five-spice powder

½ teaspoon salt

⅛ teaspoon black pepper

2 teaspoons vegetable oil, divided

1 pound salmon steaks

8 ounces fresh baby spinach leaves (about 8 cups lightly packed)

2 cloves garlic, minced

1 Combine lime peel, lime juice, ginger, five-spice powder, salt, pepper and 1 teaspoon oil in 2-quart dish. Add salmon; turn to coat. Cover; refrigerate 2 to 3 hours.

2 Combine spinach, garlic and remaining 1 teaspoon oil in 3-quart microwavable dish; toss. Cover; microwave on HIGH 2 minutes or until spinach is wilted. Drain; keep warm.

3 Meanwhile, oil grid and prepare grill for direct cooking over medium-high heat.

4 Remove salmon from marinade. Place on grid. Brush salmon with marinade. Grill salmon, covered, 4 minutes. Turn salmon; brush with marinade and grill 4 minutes or until fish just begins to flake when tested with fork. Discard remaining marinade. Serve over spinach.

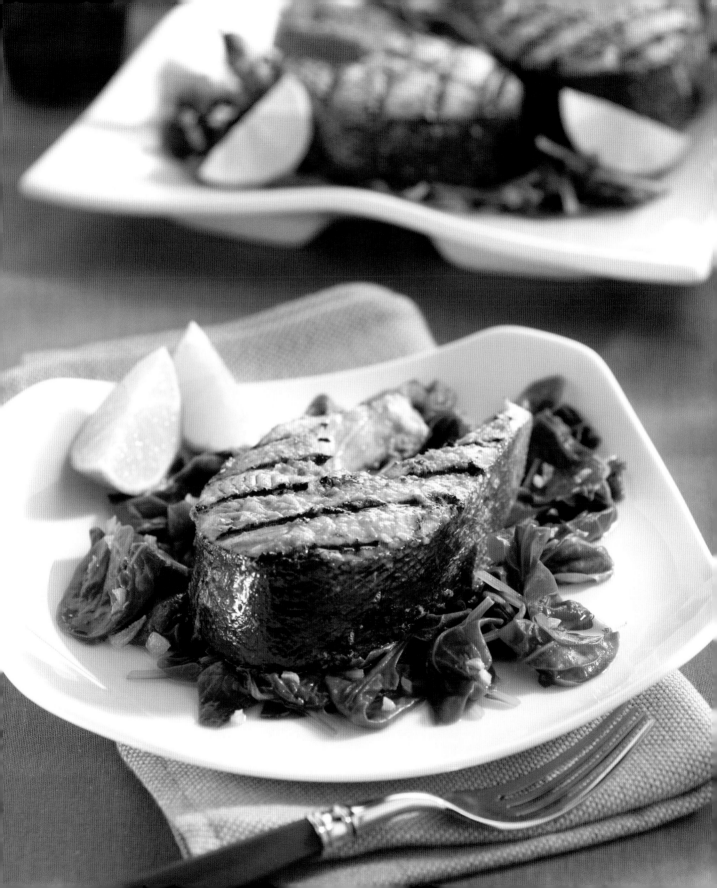

Baked Fish with Tomatoes and Herbs

NUTRIENTS PER SERVING

CALORIES
150

TOTAL FAT
4g

SATURATED FAT
1g

CHOLESTEROL
42mg

SODIUM
360mg

CARBOHYDRATE
4g

DIETARY FIBER
1g

PROTEIN
24g

MAKES 4 SERVINGS

4 lean white fish fillets (about 1 pound), such as orange roughy or sole

2 tablespoons plus 2 teaspoons lemon juice, divided

½ teaspoon paprika

1 cup finely chopped seeded tomatoes

2 tablespoons capers, rinsed and drained

2 tablespoons finely chopped fresh parsley

1½ teaspoons dried basil

2 teaspoons olive oil

¼ teaspoon salt

1 Preheat oven to 350°F. Spray 12×8-inch baking dish with nonstick cooking spray.

2 Arrange fish fillets in prepared baking dish; drizzle 2 tablespoons lemon juice over fillets and sprinkle with paprika. Cover with foil; bake 18 minutes or until fish is opaque in center and flakes easily when tested with fork.

3 Meanwhile, combine tomatoes, capers, parsley, remaining 2 teaspoons lemon juice, basil, oil and salt in medium saucepan. Bring to a boil over high heat. Reduce heat; simmer 2 minutes. Serve with fish.

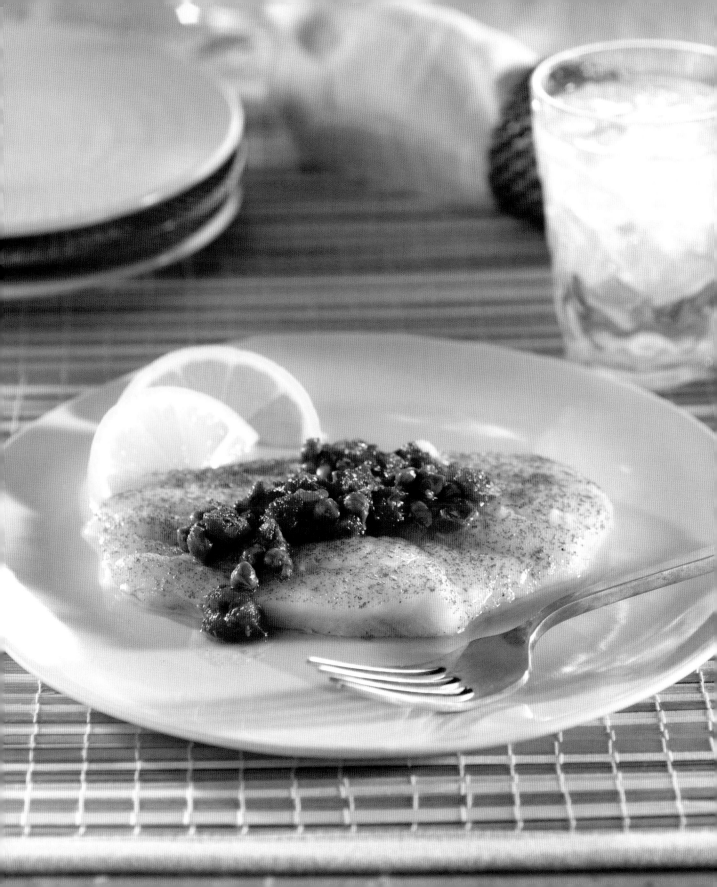

Pan-Seared Halibut Steaks with Avocado Salsa

MAKES 4 SERVINGS

4 tablespoons chipotle salsa, divided

½ teaspoon salt, divided

4 small (4 to 5 ounces) *or* 2 large (8 to 10 ounces) halibut steaks, cut ¾ inch thick

½ cup diced tomato

½ ripe avocado, diced

2 tablespoons chopped fresh cilantro (optional)

1 Combine 2 tablespoons salsa and ¼ teaspoon salt in small bowl; spread over both sides of halibut.

2 Heat large nonstick skillet over medium heat. Add halibut; cook 4 to 5 minutes per side or until fish is opaque in center.

3 Meanwhile, combine remaining 2 tablespoons salsa, ¼ teaspoon salt, tomato, avocado and cilantro, if desired, in small bowl; mix well. Serve with fish.

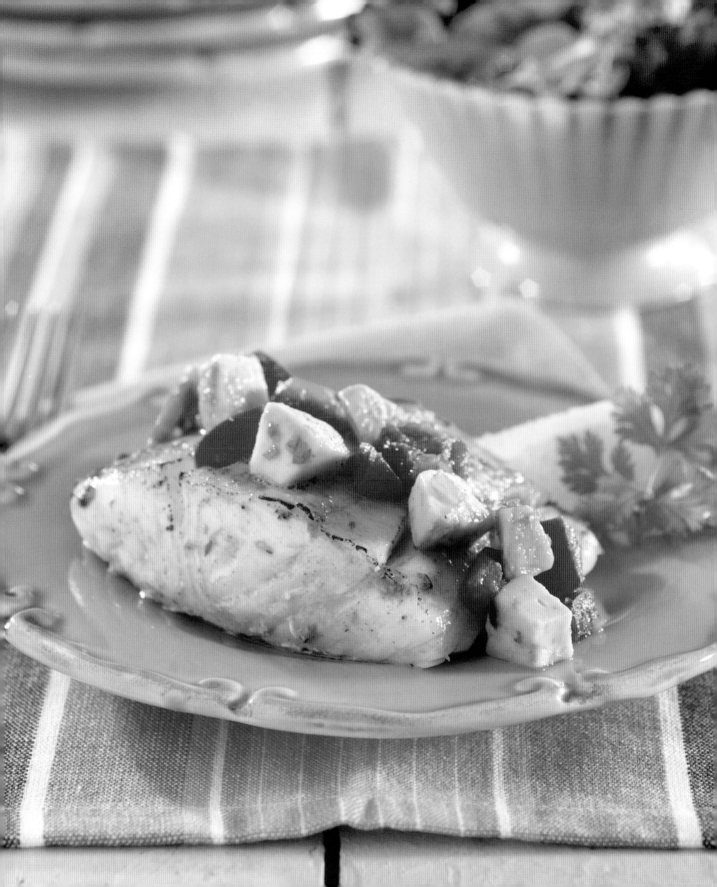

Spicy Thai Shrimp Soup

MAKES 4 SERVINGS

1 tablespoon vegetable oil

1 pound medium raw shrimp, peeled and deveined, shells reserved

1 jalapeño pepper, cut into slivers

1 tablespoon paprika

¼ teaspoon ground red pepper

4 cans (about 14 ounces each) chicken broth

1 (½-inch) strip *each* lemon and lime peel

1 can (15 ounces) straw mushrooms, drained

Juice of 1 lemon

Juice of 1 lime

2 tablespoons soy sauce

1 red Thai pepper or red jalapeño pepper *or* ¼ small red bell pepper, cut into strips

¼ cup fresh cilantro leaves

1 Heat large skillet or wok over medium-high heat 1 minute. Add oil; heat 30 seconds. Add shrimp and jalapeño; stir-fry 1 minute. Add paprika and ground red pepper; stir-fry 1 minute or until shrimp are pink and opaque. Transfer shrimp mixture to medium bowl.

2 Add shrimp shells to skillet; cook and stir 30 seconds. Add broth and lemon and lime peels; bring to a boil. Reduce heat to low; cover and simmer 15 minutes.

3 Remove and discard shells and peels with slotted spoon. Add mushrooms and shrimp mixture to broth; bring to a boil over medium heat. Stir in lemon and lime juices, soy sauce and Thai pepper; cook until heated through. Ladle soup into bowls. Sprinkle with cilantro. Serve immediately.

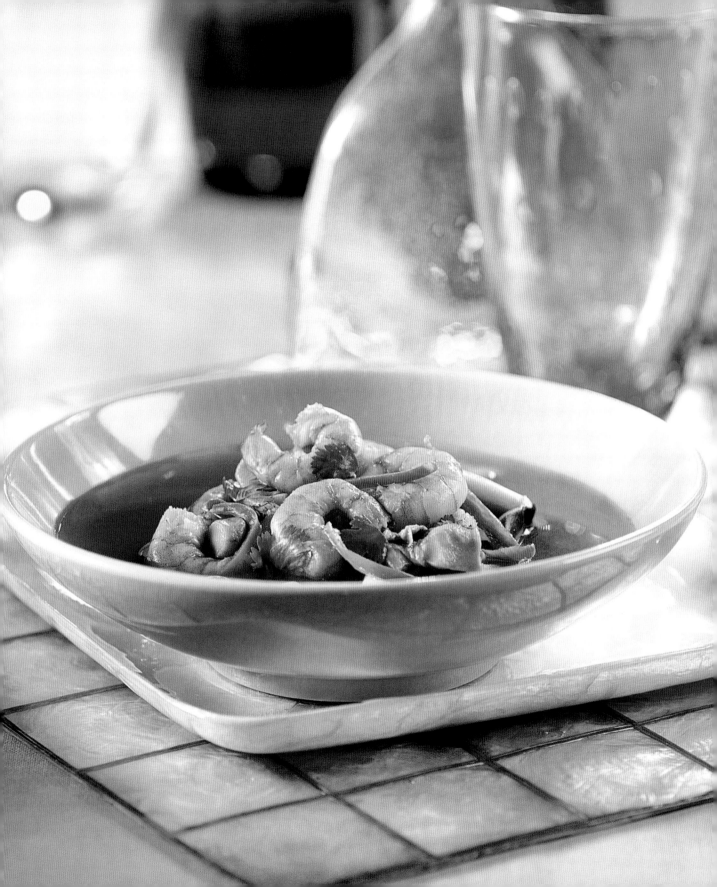

Broiled Orange Roughy with Green Peppercorn Sauce

MAKES 4 SERVINGS

1 cup loosely packed cilantro leaves

2 tablespoons dry white wine

2 tablespoons Dijon mustard

½ teaspoon green peppercorns, rinsed, drained

4 orange roughy fillets (about 6 ounces each)

1 Preheat broiler. Position oven rack about 4 inches from heat source.

2 Combine cilantro, wine, mustard and peppercorns in food processor or blender; process until well blended.

3 Place fish in shallow baking pan; top with sauce.

4 Broil 10 minutes or until fish flakes easily when tested with fork.

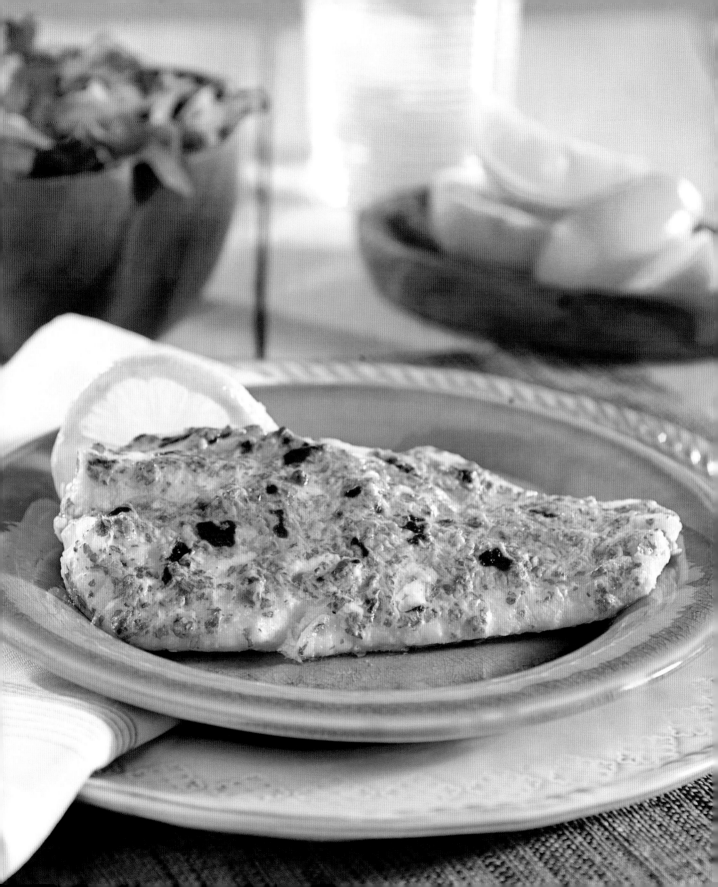

Marinated Mussels on the Half Shell

MAKES 6 SERVINGS

½ cup Tomatillo Salsa (recipe follows)

36 mussels or small hard-shell clams

Boiling water

1 tablespoon olive oil

1 tablespoon lime juice

Salt

1 Prepare Tomatillo Salsa.

2 Scrub mussels under cold water with stiff brush; discard any with open shells or with shells that do not close when tapped. Pull out and discard brown, hairlike beards. Arrange half of mussels in large skillet; pour in boiling water to depth of about ½ inch. Cover and simmer over medium heat 5 to 8 minutes or until shells open. As their shells open, remove mussels with slotted spoon; set aside to cool. Discard any unopened mussels. Repeat with remaining mussels.

3 Remove mussels from shells with small knife. Separate shells; save half. Cover shells and refrigerate. Combine Tomatillo Salsa, oil and lime juice in large bowl. Add mussels; stir to coat. Season with salt to taste. Cover and refrigerate up to 24 hours.

4 Remove mussels from marinade; place one in each shell. Arrange on platter. Spoon any remaining marinade over mussels.

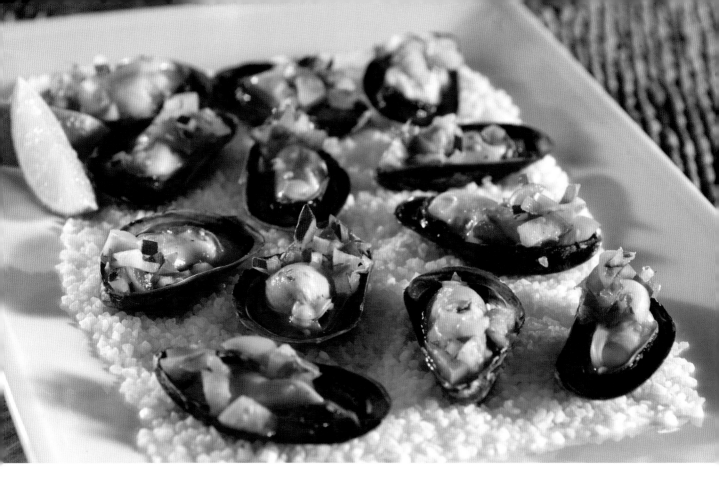

Tomatillo Salsa

MAKES ABOUT 1½ CUPS

- 1 pound tomatillos (about 12 large) *or* 1 can (13 ounces) tomatillos
- ½ cup finely chopped red onion
- ¼ cup coarsely chopped fresh cilantro
- 2 fresh jalapeño or serrano peppers, stemmed, seeded and minced
- 1 tablespoon lime juice
- 1 teaspoon olive oil
- ½ teaspoon salt

1 For fresh tomatillos, remove papery husks; wash tomatillos and finely chop. For canned tomatillos, drain and coarsely chop.

2 Combine tomatillos, onion, cilantro, jalapeño, lime juice, oil and salt in medium bowl. Cover and refrigerate 1 hour or up to 3 days for flavors to blend.

Spaghetti Squash with Shrimp and Veggies

MAKES 6 SERVINGS

NUTRIENTS PER SERVING

CALORIES
180

TOTAL FAT
8g

SATURATED FAT
1g

CHOLESTEROL
115mg

SODIUM
490mg

CARBOHYDRATE
10g

DIETARY FIBER
3g

PROTEIN
17g

1 spaghetti squash (1 pound)

4 cups fresh baby spinach

1 orange or red bell pepper, cut into 1-inch squares

½ cup julienned sun-dried tomatoes (not packed in oil)

3 tablespoons prepared pesto

2 tablespoons olive oil

½ teaspoon salt

12 ounces cooked medium shrimp

¼ cup grated Parmesan cheese (optional)

SLOW COOKER DIRECTIONS

1 Pierce squash evenly 10 times with knife. Place squash in slow cooker; add 1 inch water. Cover; cook on HIGH 2½ hours. Remove squash to large cutting board; let stand until cool enough to handle.

2 Meanwhile, pour out all but 2 tablespoons of water from slow cooker. Add spinach, bell pepper, tomatoes, pesto, oil and salt; stir to blend. Cover; cook on HIGH 5 minutes.

3 Cut squash in half lengthwise. Remove and discard seeds and fibers. Scoop pulp into shreds; return to slow cooker. Toss well with spinach mixture; place shrimp on top. Cover; cook 15 to 20 minutes or until shrimp are heated through. Serve with cheese, if desired.

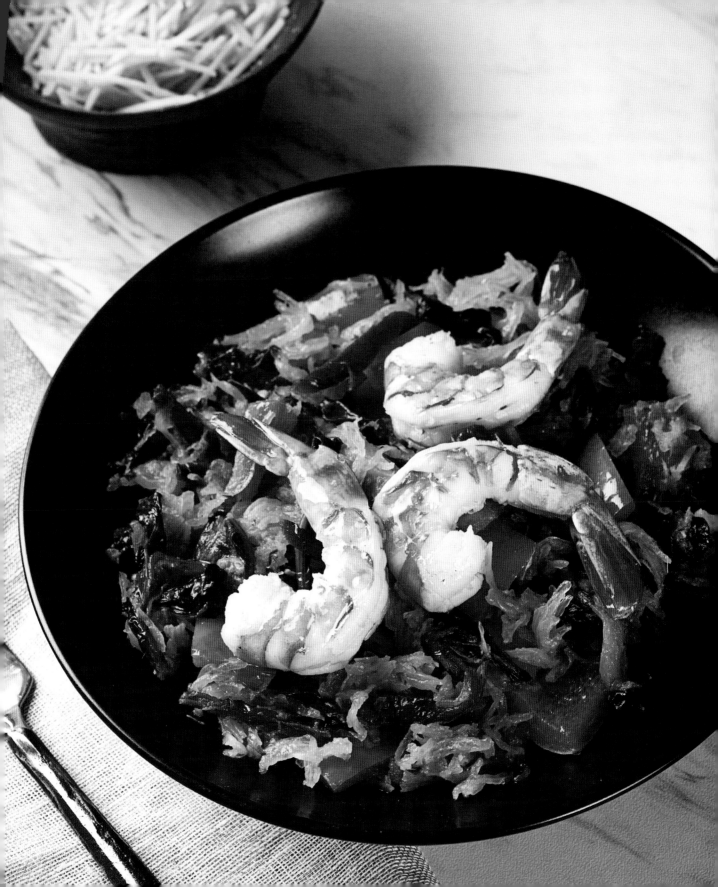

Simmering Fondue

MAKES 4 SERVINGS

4 cans (about 14 ounces each) reduced-sodium chicken broth

½ cup dry white wine

1 tablespoon chopped fresh parsley

1 teaspoon minced garlic

½ teaspoon dried thyme

½ teaspoon dried rosemary

1 pound medium raw shrimp, peeled and deveined

8 ounces beef tenderloin steaks, cut into thin slices

8 ounces lamb loin, cut into thin slices

2 cups sliced mushrooms (optional)

2 cups sliced carrots (optional)

2 cups broccoli florets (optional)

1 Combine broth, wine, parsley, garlic, thyme and rosemary in large saucepan. Bring to a boil over high heat. Remove from heat; strain broth into electric wok. Return to a simmer over high heat.

2 Thread any combination of shrimp, meat and desired vegetables onto bamboo skewer or use fondue fork. Cook in broth 2 to 3 minutes.

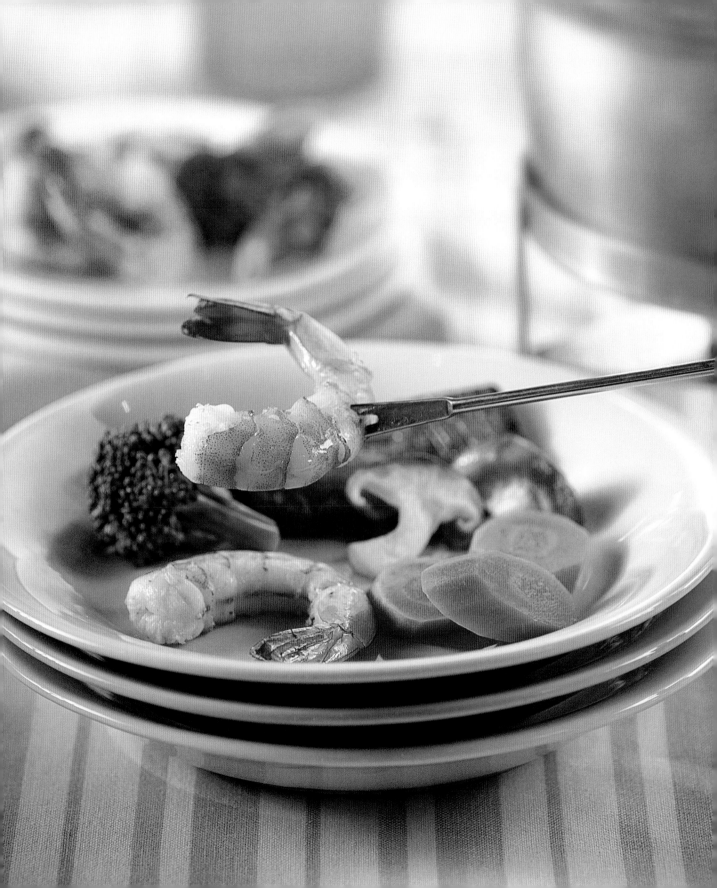

VEGETABLES AND SIDES

Asparagus with Goat Cheese Sauce

MAKES 4 TO 6 SERVINGS

1 pound asparagus, trimmed	¼ cup dry white wine
1 package (3½ ounces) goat cheese	2 cloves garlic, minced
¾ cup chicken broth	2 tablespoons chopped fresh chives

1 Steam asparagus 3 to 5 minutes or until crisp-tender.

2 Meanwhile for sauce, mash cheese in medium nonstick skillet. Stir in broth, wine and garlic. Simmer over medium heat 8 to 10 minutes or until desired thickness, stirring frequently. Fold in chives; serve immediately over asparagus.

NUTRIENTS PER SERVING

CALORIES
135

TOTAL FAT
8g

SATURATED FAT
5g

CHOLESTEROL
20mg

SODIUM
319mg

CARBOHYDRATE
7g

DIETARY FIBER
2g

PROTEIN
8g

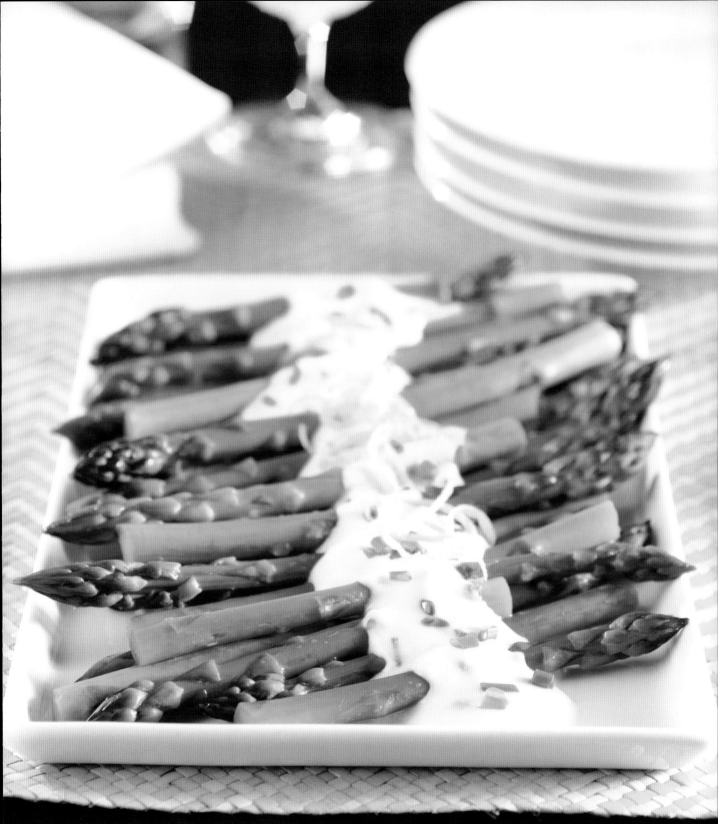

Mexican-Style Spinach

MAKES 6 SERVINGS

2 packages (16 ounces each) frozen spinach leaves

1 tablespoon canola oil

1 onion, chopped

1 clove garlic, minced

2 Anaheim chiles, toasted, peeled and minced

3 fresh tomatillos, toasted,* husks removed and chopped

Sour cream (optional)

To toast fresh tomatillos, preheat heavy skillet over medium heat. Leaving papery husks on, toast tomatillos, turning often, about 10 minutes or until husks are brown and interior flesh is soft. Remove from heat. When cool enough to handle, remove and discard husks.

SLOW COOKER DIRECTIONS

1 Place frozen spinach in slow cooker.

2 Heat oil in large skillet over medium heat. Add onion and garlic; cook and stir about 5 minutes or until onion is softened. Add chiles and tomatillos; cook and stir 2 to 3 minutes. Transfer mixture to slow cooker. Cover; cook on LOW 4 to 6 hours. Stir before serving. Serve with sour cream, if desired.

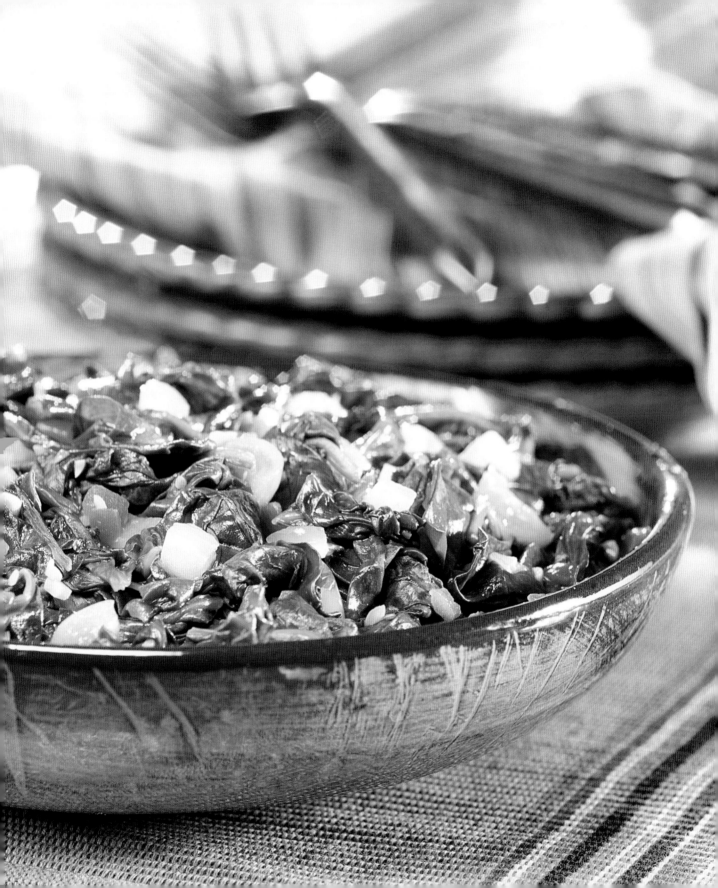

Grilled Feta with Peppers

MAKES 8 SERVINGS

¼ cup thinly sliced sweet onion

1 package (8 ounces) chunk feta cheese, sliced in half horizontally

¼ cup thinly sliced green bell pepper

¼ cup thinly sliced red bell pepper

½ teaspoon dried oregano

¼ teaspoon garlic pepper or black pepper

NUTRIENTS PER SERVING

CALORIES
70

TOTAL FAT
5g

SATURATED FAT
3g

CHOLESTEROL
10mg

SODIUM
360mg

CARBOHYDRATE
2g

DIETARY FIBER
0g

PROTEIN
5g

1 Prepare grill for direct cooking. Spray 14-inch-long sheet of foil with nonstick cooking spray. Place onion slices in center of foil and top with feta slices. Sprinkle with bell pepper slices, oregano and garlic pepper.

2 Seal foil using Drugstore Wrap technique (see below). Place foil packet on grid upside down. Grill, covered, over medium-high heat 15 minutes. Turn packet over; grill 15 minutes.

3 Open packet carefully and serve immediately.

DRUGSTORE WRAP

Bring two long sides of foil together above the food; fold down in a series of locked folds, allowing for heat circulation and expansion. Fold short ends up and over again. Press folds firmly to seal the foil packet.

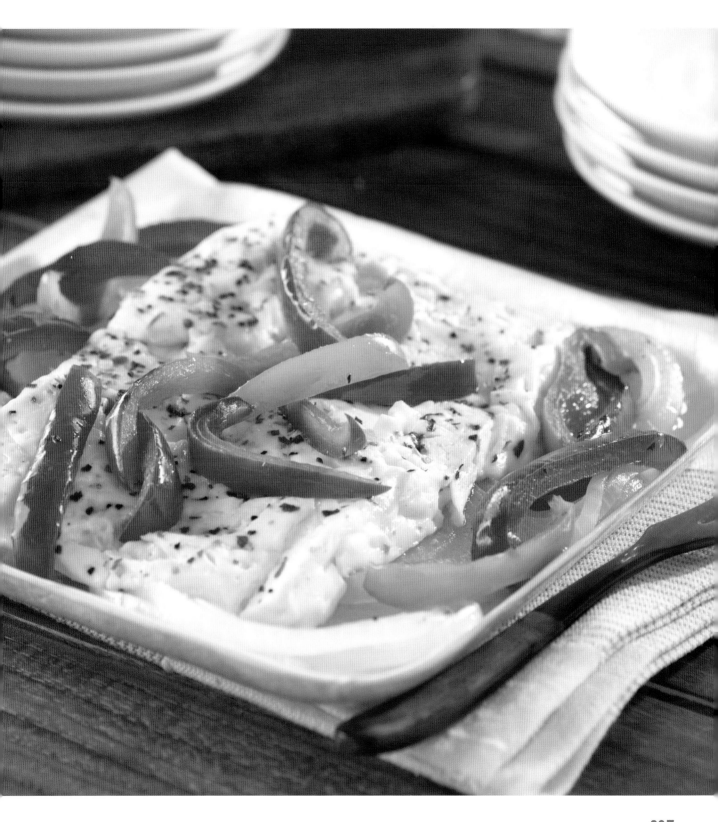

Mashed Cauliflower

MAKES 6 SERVINGS

2 heads cauliflower (8 cups florets)

1 tablespoon butter

1 tablespoon half-and-half, whole milk or buttermilk

Salt

1 Break cauliflower into equal-size florets. Place in large saucepan; add about 2 inches of water. Simmer over medium heat 20 to 25 minutes or until cauliflower is very tender and falling apart. (Check occasionally to make sure there is enough water to prevent burning; add water if necessary.) Drain well.

2 Place cooked cauliflower in food processor or blender. Process until almost smooth. Add butter. Process until smooth, adding cream as needed to reach desired consistency. Season with salt to taste.

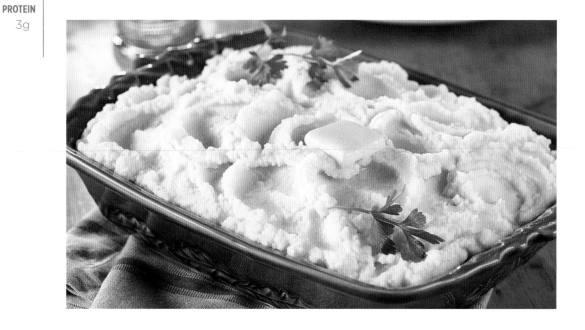

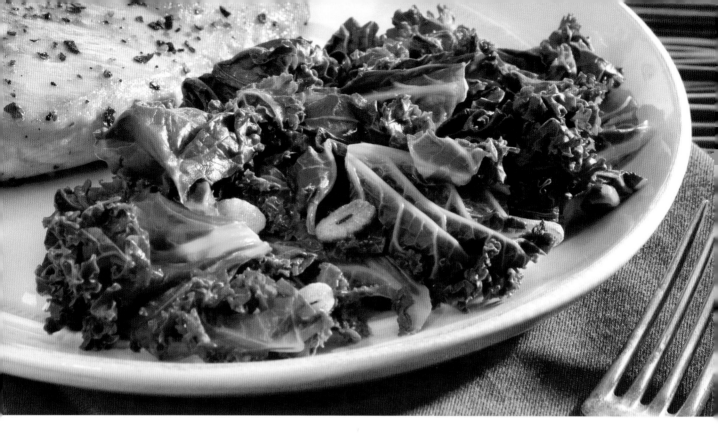

Kale with Caramelized Garlic

MAKES 8 SERVINGS

NUTRIENTS
PER SERVING

CALORIES
62

TOTAL FAT
2g

SATURATED FAT
0g

CHOLESTEROL
0mg

SODIUM
180mg

CARBOHYDRATE
10g

DIETARY FIBER
2g

PROTEIN
3g

1½ pounds fresh kale, tough stems removed and discarded, leaves thinly sliced (16 cups)

2 cups water

1 tablespoon olive oil

8 cloves garlic, thinly sliced

1 teaspoon red wine vinegar

¼ teaspoon salt

⅛ to ¼ teaspoon red pepper flakes

1 Place kale and water in large saucepan; bring to a boil over medium-high heat. Cover and cook 6 to 8 minutes or until kale is tender but still bright green. Drain in colander.

2 Meanwhile, heat oil in large nonstick skillet over medium heat. Add garlic; cook and stir 4 minutes or until garlic is golden brown, being careful not to allow garlic to burn. Add kale, vinegar, salt and red pepper flakes; cook and stir until heated through.

Zoodles in Tomato Sauce

MAKES 8 SERVINGS

NUTRIENTS
PER SERVING

CALORIES
70

TOTAL FAT
3g

SATURATED FAT
1g

CHOLESTEROL
3mg

SODIUM
360mg

CARBOHYDRATE
8g

DIETARY FIBER
3g

PROTEIN
4g

3 teaspoons olive oil, divided

2 cloves garlic

1 tablespoon tomato paste

1 can (28 ounces) whole tomatoes

1 teaspoon dried oregano

½ teaspoon salt

2 large zucchini (about 16 ounces each), ends trimmed, cut into 3-inch pieces

¼ cup shredded Parmesan cheese

1 Heat 2 teaspoons oil in medium saucepan over medium heat. Add garlic; cook 1 minute or until fragrant but not browned. Stir in tomato paste; cook 30 seconds, stirring constantly. Add tomatoes with juice, oregano and salt; break up tomatoes with wooden spoon. Bring to a simmer. Reduce heat; cook 30 minutes or until thickened.

2 Meanwhile, spiral zucchini with fine spiral blade. Heat remaining 1 teaspoon oil in large skillet over medium-high heat. Add zucchini; cook 4 to 5 minutes or until tender, stirring frequently. Transfer to serving plates; top with tomato sauce and Parmesan cheese, if desired.

NOTE

If you don't have a spiralizer, cut the zucchini into ribbons with a mandoline or sharp knife. Or for small wedges that mimic a small pasta shape, cut it lengthwise into quarters and then thinly slice it crosswise.

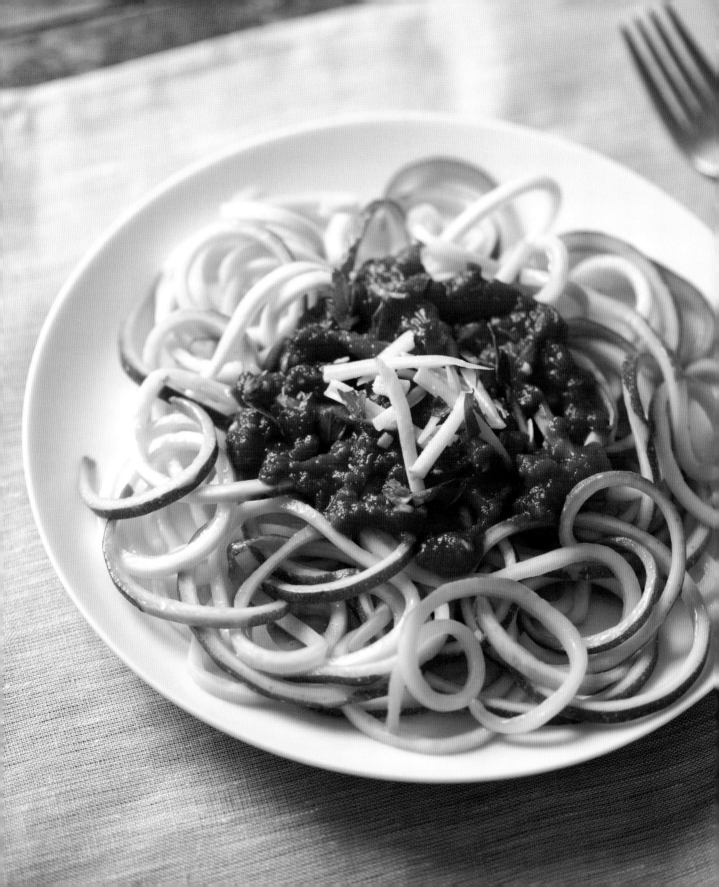

Grilled Sesame Asparagus

MAKES 4 SERVINGS

Nonstick cooking spray

1 pound medium asparagus spears (about 20), trimmed

1 tablespoon sesame seeds

2 to 3 teaspoons balsamic vinegar

¼ teaspoon salt

¼ teaspoon black pepper

1 Spray grid with cooking spray. Prepare grill for direct cooking.

2 Place asparagus on baking sheet; spray lightly with cooking spray. Sprinkle with the sesame seeds; roll to coat.

3 Place asparagus on grid. Grill, uncovered, 4 to 6 minutes or until asparagus begins to brown, turning once.

4 Transfer asparagus to serving dish. Sprinkle with vinegar, salt and pepper.

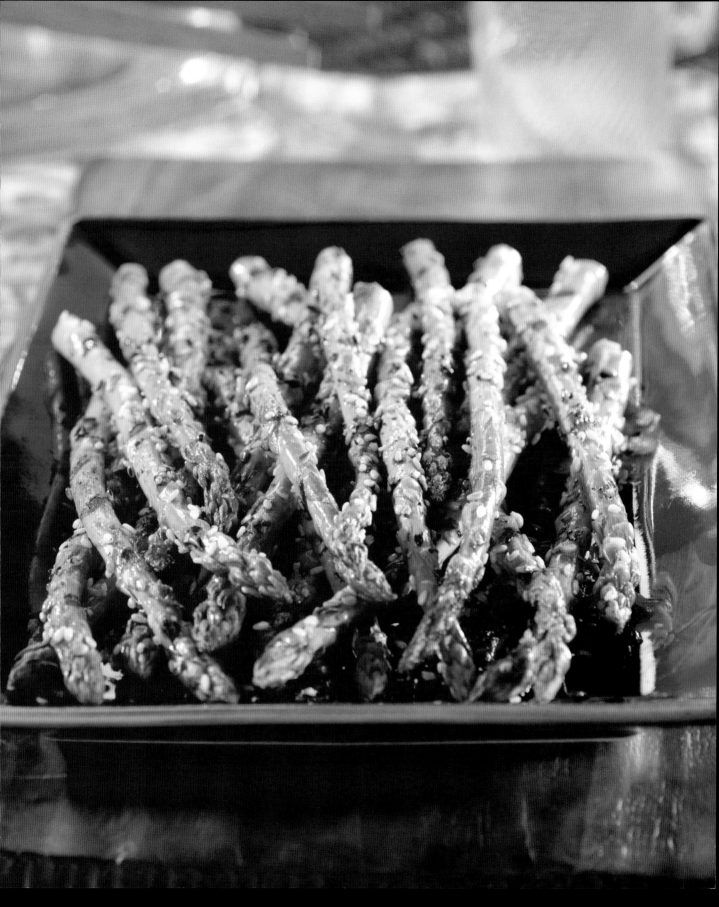

Colorful Coleslaw

MAKES 8 SERVINGS

¼ head green cabbage, shredded or thinly sliced

¼ head red cabbage, shredded or thinly sliced

1 small yellow or orange bell pepper, thinly sliced

1 small jicama, peeled and julienned

¼ cup thinly sliced green onions

2 tablespoons chopped fresh cilantro

¼ cup vegetable oil

¼ cup fresh lime juice

1 teaspoon salt

⅛ teaspoon black pepper

1 Combine cabbage, bell pepper, jicama, green onions and cilantro in large bowl.

2 Whisk oil, lime juice, salt and black pepper in small bowl until well blended. Pour over vegetables; toss to coat. Cover and refrigerate 2 to 6 hours for flavors to blend.

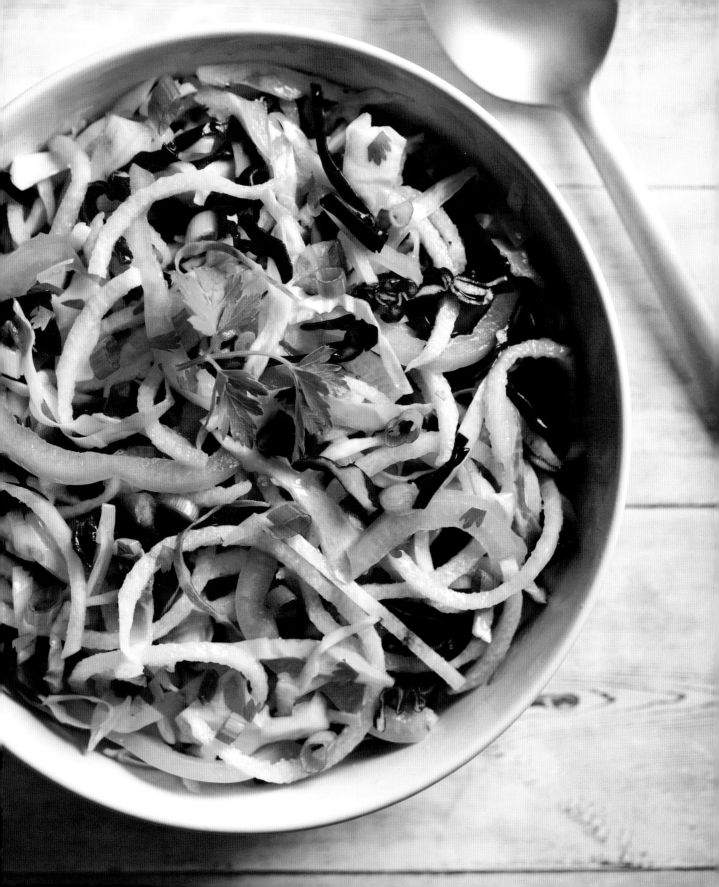

Creamy Parmesan Spinach

MAKES 6 SERVINGS (½ CUP EACH)

2 tablespoons butter, divided

1 cup finely chopped yellow onion

1 package (10 ounces) fresh spinach leaves

3 ounces cream cheese, diced

½ teaspoon garlic powder

¼ teaspoon ground nutmeg

¼ teaspoon black pepper

⅛ teaspoon salt

2 tablespoons grated Parmesan, pecorino or Monterey Jack cheese

1 Melt 1 tablespoon butter in large skillet over medium-high heat. Add onion; cook and stir 4 minutes or until translucent.

2 Add half of spinach; cook and stir 2 minutes or just until wilted. Transfer to medium bowl. Repeat with remaining 1 tablespoon butter and spinach.

3 Add reserved spinach to skillet. Add cream cheese, garlic powder, nutmeg, pepper and salt; cook and stir until cheese has completely melted. Sprinkle with Parmesan cheese; serve immediately.

VARIATION

For a thinner consistency, add 2 to 3 tablespoons milk before adding the Parmesan cheese.

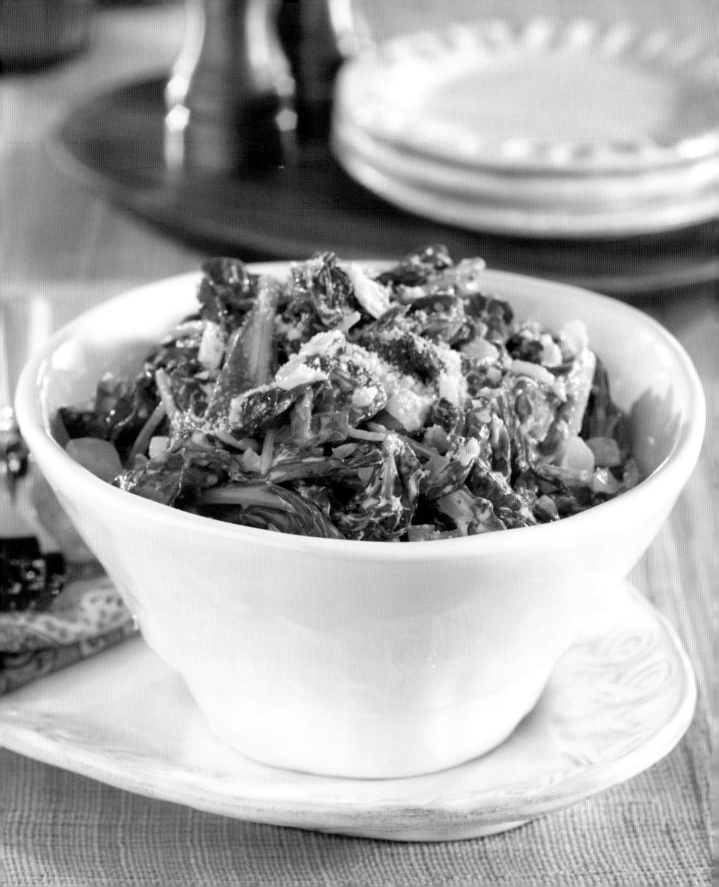

Sautéed Swiss Chard

MAKES 4 SERVINGS

1 large bunch Swiss chard or kale (about 1 pound)

1 tablespoon olive oil

3 cloves garlic, minced

¾ teaspoon salt

¼ teaspoon black pepper

1 tablespoon balsamic vinegar (optional)

¼ cup pine nuts, toasted*

To toast pine nuts, spread in single layer in heavy skillet. Cook and stir over medium heat 1 to 2 minutes or until nuts are lightly browned, stirring frequently.

1 Rinse chard in cold water; shake off excess water but do not dry. Finely chop stems and coarsely chop leaves.

2 Heat oil in large saucepan or Dutch oven over medium heat. Add garlic; cook and stir 2 minutes. Add chard, salt and pepper. Cover; cook 2 minutes or until chard begins to wilt. Uncover; cook and stir about 5 minutes or until chard is evenly wilted.

3 Stir in vinegar, if desired. Sprinkle with pine nuts just before serving.

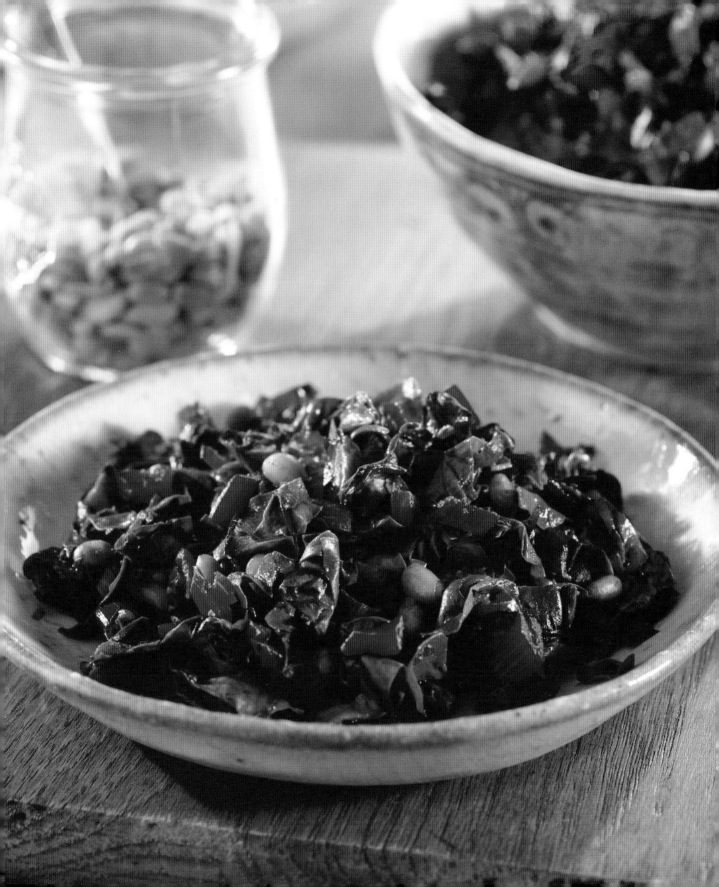

Sautéed Kale with Mushrooms and Bacon

NUTRIENTS PER SERVING

CALORIES
90

TOTAL FAT
4g

SATURATED FAT
1g

CHOLESTEROL
5mg

SODIUM
90mg

CARBOHYDRATE
11g

DIETARY FIBER
3g

PROTEIN
4g

MAKES 4 SERVINGS

1 slice bacon, chopped

½ cup sliced shallots

1 package (4 ounces) sliced mixed exotic mushrooms *or* 8 ounces cremini mushrooms, sliced

10 cups loosely packed torn fresh kale leaves (about 8 ounces),* stems removed

2 tablespoons water

½ teaspoon black pepper

*Buy loose kale leaves or look for 16 ounce bags of ready-to-cook fresh kale leaves in the produce section of the supermarket

1 Cook bacon in large heavy skillet over medium heat 5 minutes. Add shallots; cook and stir 3 minutes. Add mushrooms; cook and stir 8 minutes.

2 Add kale and water; cover and cook 5 minutes. Uncover; cook and stir 5 minutes or until kale is crisp-tender. Season with pepper.

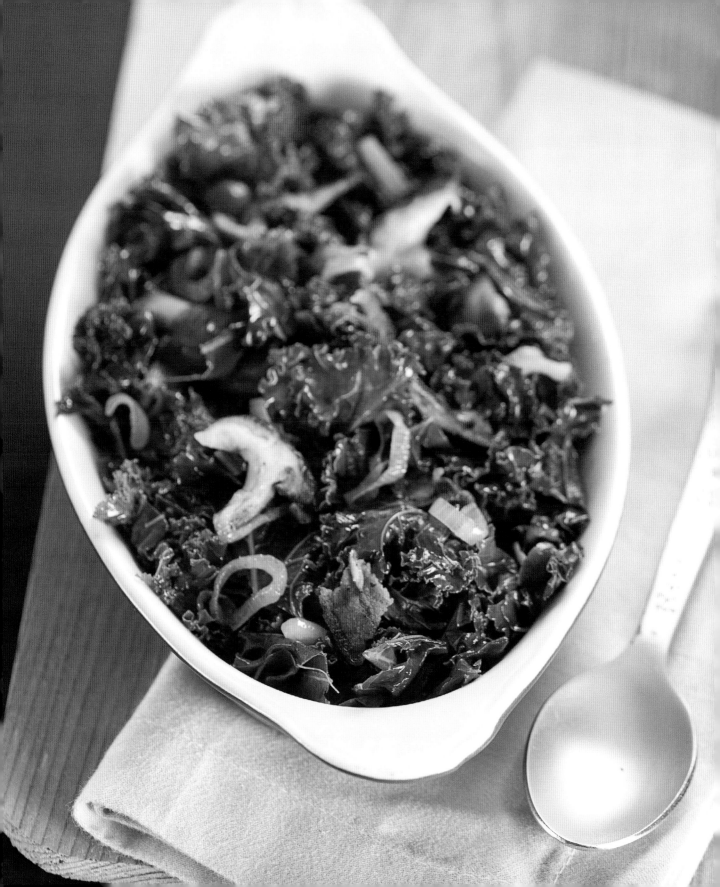

METRIC CONVERSION CHART

VOLUME MEASUREMENTS (dry)

1/8 teaspoon = 0.5 mL
1/4 teaspoon = 1 mL
1/2 teaspoon = 2 mL
3/4 teaspoon = 4 mL
1 teaspoon = 5 mL
1 tablespoon = 15 mL
2 tablespoons = 30 mL
1/4 cup = 60 mL
1/3 cup = 75 mL
1/2 cup = 125 mL
2/3 cup = 150 mL
3/4 cup = 175 mL
1 cup = 250 mL
2 cups = 1 pint = 500 mL
3 cups = 750 mL
4 cups = 1 quart = 1 L

VOLUME MEASUREMENTS (fluid)

1 fluid ounce (2 tablespoons) = 30 mL
4 fluid ounces (1/2 cup) = 125 mL
8 fluid ounces (1 cup) = 250 mL
12 fluid ounces (1 1/2 cups) = 375 mL
16 fluid ounces (2 cups) = 500 mL

WEIGHTS (mass)

1/2 ounce = 15 g
1 ounce = 30 g
3 ounces = 90 g
4 ounces = 120 g
8 ounces = 225 g
10 ounces = 285 g
12 ounces = 360 g
16 ounces = 1 pound = 450 g

DIMENSIONS

1/16 inch = 2 mm
1/8 inch = 3 mm
1/4 inch = 6 mm
1/2 inch = 1.5 cm
3/4 inch = 2 cm
1 inch = 2.5 cm

OVEN TEMPERATURES

250°F = 120°C
275°F = 140°C
300°F = 150°C
325°F = 160°C
350°F = 180°C
375°F = 190°C
400°F = 200°C
425°F = 220°C
450°F = 230°C

BAKING PAN SIZES

Utensil	Size in Inches/Quarts	Metric Volume	Size in Centimeters
Baking or Cake Pan (square or rectangular)	8×8×2	2 L	20×20×5
	9×9×2	2.5 L	23×23×5
	12×8×2	3 L	30×20×5
	13×9×2	3.5 L	33×23×5
Loaf Pan	8×4×3	1.5 L	20×10×7
	9×5×3	2 L	23×13×7
Round Layer Cake Pan	8×1½	1.2 L	20×4
	9×1½	1.5 L	23×4
Pie Plate	8×1¼	750 mL	20×3
	9×1¼	1 L	23×3
Baking Dish or Casserole	1 quart	1 L	—
	1½ quart	1.5 L	—
	2 quart	2 L	—